MW01114934

Backstage Passes:
An Anthology of Rock and Roll Erotica
from the Pages of Blue Blood

edited by Amelia G

Backstage Passes: An Anthology of Rock and Roll Erotica from the Pages of Blue Blood

Copyright © 2010 by Amelia G
All rights reserved.
ISBN 978-0-9846053-1-6
Ebook format is ISBN 978-0-9846053-2-3
Manufactured in the United States of America.
Published by Blue Blood CBLT, 8033 Sunset Blvd #4500, West Hollywood, CA 90046, USA. Originally published in slightly different form by Masquerade Rhinoceros, New York, NY in 1996 under ISBN 1-56333-438-0.

Library of Congress Control Number 2010931242

"Chanel No. 5" by Johnny Chen. Copyright © 1992 by Johnny Chen. Published originally by CBLT in *Blue Blood #1*. Reprinted by permission of CBLT and the author.

"New Introduction" by Amelia G. Copyright © 2010 by Amelia G. An original piece published by permission of the author.

"Preface" and story introductions by Amelia G. Copyright © 1995 by Amelia G. Original pieces published by permission of the author with the exception of part of the Poppy Z. Brite bio which was published originally in *Blue Blood #3* and is reprinted by permission of CBLT.

"When Enter Came" by John Shirley. Copyright © 1990 by John Shirley. Published originally first in *Yellow Silk #33*, 1990 and then in *The Exploded Heart*, ed. Steve Brown,

Eyeball Books, Ashville, 1996. Reprinted by permission of Lily Pond, Steve Brown and the author.

"Sticky Fingers" by Thomas S. Roche. Copyright © 1995 by Thomas S. Roche. An original piece published by permission of the author.

"Temporary Assignment" by Will Judy. Copyright © 1995 by Will Judy. An original piece published by permission of the author.

"Rock Steady" by Cecilia Tan. Copyright © 1995 by Cecilia Tan. An original piece published by permission of the author.

"Demon Lover" by Nancy A. Collins. Copyright © 1991 by Nancy A. Collins. Published originally by CBLT in *Blue Blood #2*. An earlier version of this story was published in *Hotter Blood*, ed. Jeff Gelb and Michael Garrett, Pocket Books, New York, 1991. Reprinted by permission of the author.

"Music of My Damnation" by William Spencer-Hale. Copyright © 1993 by William Spencer-Hale. Published originally by CBLT in *Blue Blood #3*. Reprinted by permission of CBLT and the author.

"Bodie" by Sèphera Girón. Copyright © 1995 by Sèphera Girón. An original piece published by permission of the author.

"Accept No Substitutes" by Sarah McKinley Oakes. Copyright © 1995 by Sarah McKinley Oakes. An original piece published by permission of the author.

"Dreamgirl" by Amelia G. Copyright © 1995 by Amelia G. An original piece published by permission of the author.

"Not Another Groupie" by Andrew Green•berg. Copyright © 1995 by Andrew Greenberg. An original piece published by permission of the author.

"To An Excellent Slave" by L. Copyright © 1992 by CBLT. Published originally by CBLT in *Blue Blood #1*. Reprinted by permission of CBLT.

"The Ceremony of Loneliness" by Althea Morin. Copyright © 1994 by Althea Morin. Published originally by CBLT in *Blue Blood #4*. Reprinted by permission of CBLT.

"Private" by t. d. k. Copyright © 1992 by CBLT. Published originally by CBLT in *Blue Blood #1*. Reprinted by permission of CBLT and the author.

"Lacerations" by Yon Von Faust. Copyright © 1993 by Yon Von Faust. Published originally by CBLT in *Blue Blood #2*. Reprinted by permission of CBLT and the author.

"Pipe Dreams" by Shariann Lewitt. Copyright © 1992 by S. N. Lewitt. Published originally by CBLT in *Blue Blood #5*. An earlier version of this story was published first in *All Hallows Eve*, ed. Mary Elizabeth Allen, Walker, New York, 1992 and then in *Sex Magick*, ed. Cecilia Tan, Circlet Press, Boston, 1994. Reprinted by permission of the author.

"America" by Poppy Z. Brite. Copyright © 1995 by Poppy Z. Brite. An original piece published by permission of the author.

Backstage Passes:

An Anthology of Rock and Roll Erotica
from the Pages of Blue Blood

Chanel No. 5

by Johnny Chen

Brutal gigs in Screw City.
Thrash-punk chicks . . .
Night shades,
Dog-gnawed neon hair,
Finger-painted faces,
Kinky jewelry.
Raunchy nylon strides
slink on sharp heels.
Leather whispers with lace.
Moving mouths--
Vermilion lips round on Sugar & Mints
Fruity gum smacks smoke.
Ruby tongues, wet and moist,
Lick switchblade nails
On phallic fingers--
Slashes, Flashes, Trips, Tricks.
Brusque Burlesques sweat
Chanel No. 5

New Introduction
by Amelia G

Blue Blood's Backstage Passes was first published many moons ago by Richard Kasak's Masquerade Books. The term paranormal romance wasn't being used yet, but the new generation of top notch genre fiction writers wore leather jackets, sported unusual haircuts, and wrote about sex and love and rock and roll. As well as about aliens and monsters.

In 1996, I lived in Maryland and fellow Wesleyan University alum and professional pervert Tristan Taormino had written fiction which appeared in Blue Blood magazine and she was working for Richard Kasak. Tristan and I were chatting on the phone and she asked if I'd like to do an anthology for the Masquerade Books literary imprint Rhinoceros. Of course, I was excited to do the project and got to work selecting some of the best stories which had graced the pages of Blue Blood magazine and an assortment of new work with a rock and roll erotic theme. By the time the book came out, I was living in Atlanta, Georgia and Tristan wasn't working at Masquerade any more, which meant that I didn't get to include her Blue Blood fiction in the book and I felt a bit disconnected from the process.

By the time Backstage Passes was getting rave reviews, I was sort of doing the couch tour -- as both starving writers and bands often do -- which ultimately lead to moving to California. Industrial Nation magazine gushed, "*Backstage Passes is a compilation of dynamic authors who write excellent fiction. I was charged by this book from first sentence to last. Here are 18 works of spell binding literature ... I got from this book what I needed, and recommend it*". Dirty magazine stated, "*this collection of short stories explores the connection between* lust and rock and roll, and does it rather well ... the bottom line is that it's a top-notch erotica omnibus." Redemption magazine raved, "an anthology of Rock-and-Roll Erotica that is sure to stimulate the mind, heart and other places. There is nothing like this out there ... If you like your Rock and Roll the way it was meant to be, this is a reading must. It is an erotic multisexual romp through modern music subculture, from vampire kids to heavy metal guitarists, backstage trysts ... Nothing is comparable to this compendium."

Backstage Passes did well in the traditional bookstore outlets, both the mom and pop establishments and Barnes & Noble and Borders. It was one of the few fiction anthologies selected to be distributed to every Tower Records in the world. Masquerade Books also had specialty distribution which enabled Backstage Passes to be sold at most newsstands which carried Playgirl and High Society and related magazines. After seeing used copies of the book selling on Amazon for as much as $63, I felt it was time to put Backstage Passes back into proper distribution and not just do the occasional handmade or one-off copy for a collector. I might not be able to do everything Masquerade Books could, but you hold in your hands the result of this desire.

I resisted the impulse to rewrite all the introductions for this edition. The contributors have all done so many amazing things, which I am really impressed by and feel honored that they chose to work with me. Plus, after years of involvement with the Los Angeles music scene, I feel almost embarrassed by the enthusiasm I wrote some of this with, but that's okay because I think readers will enjoy it. I'm going to keep you all updated about what the various writing contributors to Blue Blood have been up to at BlueBloodBooks.com and that site also has contributor guidelines. There is more visual contributor news at BlueBlood.com in the Contributor Pages. My personal digital abode is AmeliaG.com

Since the publication of the first edition of Backstage Passes, I've built a bit of a transmedia empire. As a company, Blue Blood packages cool content, sometimes for Blue Blood projects to publish and sometimes on a white label basis for other companies, which might need a book or web site or magazine done to their specifications. Blue Blood art director Forrest Black now manages the technology, look and feel of hundreds of sites. In partnership, he and I have photographed members of more than one hundred bands ranging from old school luminaries Taime Downe and Anthony Kiedis to superstars of tomorrow Andy LaPlegua and Adam Lambert.

Last year, I was deeply jazzed to be published in Rolling Stone. So the music does still turn me on. I hope it does it for you too.

--Amelia G, Hollywood, CA, 2010

First Edition Preface
by Amelia G

When I graduated from Wesleyan University, my parents asked me what I wanted for a graduation gift. This was peculiar in and of itself as my parents normally don't do special occasions. If they want to give a present or whatever, they just do it rather than waiting for a particular event. At any rate, after much deliberation, I finally told them that I wanted a really good black leather weekend bag.

Maybe they suspected that I wanted to drive rivets and studs into Gucci leather and use it to cart around my prodigious collection of bondage equipment. Maybe they just didn't think a weekend bag was a festive enough gift. Whatever their rationale was, what they gave me was a CD player and a few CDs.

So instead of getting a corporate job as was expected of me, I spent the next three years working as a stagehand and doing music journalism and costuming, eating Ramen noodles, and being forced to keep my leather straps and riot cuffs and X-acto kit in a bedraggled backpack. Not that any of the rock and rollers I tied up in the back of my car ever complained that they would have liked that condom or dental dam a whole lot better coming out of a more stylish carry-on.

I loved the lanky glam boys with their poofy hair and eyeliner and bondage belts they didn't know how to use. I loved the big-titted metal girls spilling out of their spandex. I loved the angry little punks with their shaved heads and multiple piercings and secret poetry. I loved the pale-skinned vampire gents who wished morphine was still in style. I loved the doe-eyed Goth girls with their jutting hipbones and melancholy romance. I loved the hipper-than-thou gearheads with their beautiful skin art and shirtless sweaty mosh pits. I was high on the music and the pheromones and the style. I craved the intensity and I was ready to come to the beat and I thought everyone else should be ready too.

So, somewhere along the line I decided to do a magazine of counterculture erotica. I called the publication Blue Blood and it just blossomed out of my lifestyle, out of the lifestyle triggered by that CD player. A little less than half of the stories in this anthology previously ran in Blue Blood.

This anthology is about the eroticism of music subcultures. And I know you like to look at freaky individuals up on that stage or across that smoky club . . . and I know you can feel the beat . . . feel it between your tensed thighs. Are you ready to rock?

--Amelia G, Gaithersburg, MD, 1995

John Shirley's main characters are nearly always sexy. Sexy in that way where you know you shouldn't want to fuck them, but you do anyway. Shirley writes successfully in a number of genres. I first came across his work in his cyberpunk (before the word was trite and played) trilogy A Song Called Youth. A Song Called Youth *is a complex near-future view which incorporates elements of pop culture rarely seen in science fiction. A lot of Shirley's more recent work is in the horror and crime noir genres, including* Wetbones *a creepy novel he did for Ziesing which explores the nature of addiction. His short story collections include* Heatseeker, New Noir, *and* The Exploded Heart. *John Shirley has fronted rock bands, written lyrics for Blue Oyster Cult, had green hair, and by all reports been in general as extreme a gutter punk as any of my unsavory pals. Oh yeah, and he was one of the two guys who wrote the screenplay for the movie version of* The Crow.

When Enter Came
by John Shirley

There was no contact. He was hard, or hard enough anyway, and he was inside her. He had his arms around her; their tongues worked expertly together. She groaned on cue, and thrust her hips to meet his. But there was no contact. The whole thing was a lifeless minuet performed by skilled dancers. It was sex for Buzz Garret and Elena Garret.

David Letterman was in the room. The TV was still on, in the background, but the sound was off. The only light in their bedroom was videolight, shape-shifting in pixel colors and shadow. Garret ejaculated, and thought of a line from a Lou Reed song: *Something flickered and was gone . . .*

Afterward, Elena went to the bathroom. He heard the faint plastic rattling that meant she was getting a prescription bottle. Taking a Xanax.

He thought: How did we get this way? Is it Elena? It's me as much as her. She's a bit more openly nasty sometimes, is all. She can't blame me for the career thing. She was in graduate school when we met; I was in a rock band, then. One that never made any money. She had the career momentum. I never asked her to give up her Physics R & D . . .

But somehow Garret became a booking agent, Elena became a housewife, set quantum physics aside for the glib comfort of astrology and mysticism; stays up late reading about the occult, never says a word to Garret about what she really believes . . .

She came back to bed. "Elena?" he asked.

"Hm?"

"What do you really believe? I mean, about what we're here for, what the universe is—all the stuff you read about."

"What the hell kind of time is this to ask me, Buzz? It's almost one-thirty in the morning, Jenny's going to come prancing in here waking us up promptly at seven—"

"Okay forget it."

"I mean, I'm too tired to get into—"

"Okay, okay."

No contact.

* * * * *

Three weeks and no further sex later.

"Come off it, Buzz, you love booking bands. It's the best job in the world except maybe astronaut, and that's quoting you," Elena said. He could tell she didn't like the direction of the conversation; she stared into the middle distance and used her weary, patronizing tone. "You're kind of young for a midlife crisis. Thirty-one. I mean, Christ."

It was all just her way of saying, Don't talk about it, it makes me nervous. Warning him that if he insisted on talking about it, there'd be a fight. They had a house to pay off, this was no time for a change in careers.

They were sitting in the back yard, in lawn chairs by the lawn table, on which the bones of T-bone steaks soaked grease through paper plates. The brick barbecue gave up a faint ghost of gray smoke. Elena and Garret: lounging in the soft California sunlight that went like an accessory with any Bay Area suburb, with this moderately pricey development in Walnut Creek. Elena was smoking a cigarette through one of those attachable filter-holders that strains the smoke to help you cut back. She chain-smoked to compensate.

He was tempted to point that out. But it would precipitate more snippiness. Pointless wrangling. He would be using it against her because he was angry . . .

Around and around in his head. Thinking, no contact,

no real contact. We could take X, maybe, like Barry recommended, the drug MDMA, supposed to get you closer to your spouse. But Garret was scared of drugs, after putting in a year in NA to get off cocaine. And he didn't know if he *wanted* to get closer to Elena. She wasn't particularly interested in him, not really. She didn't even know why he was nicknamed Buzz. She'd never asked, and probably thought it was like Buzz Aldrin. But it was short for Buzzard. Because Garret had been in one of the first west coast punk bands.

He looked around at his big yard, his barbecue, his two story pastel-blue split level house, and thought, How did I get from shrieking rhythmic obscenities under a mohawk, to *this*?

He loved the house, in his way. It was like one big baby crib for him and his kids. Being punk, by contrast, was like being a flagpole sitter. It had a limited appeal. It was not a career move. But it'd had one thing. It had contact, of sorts.

He could never go back to it, of course. But maybe there was some other kind of deep contact to be had . . .

Louis and Birdy were over by the rose bushes playing He-Man and She-Ra. They had the prop swords, bought at Toys-R-Us. Louis was being She-Ra, which irritated Elena, made her worry about the boy's sexual identity. "Oh He-Man," four year old Louis was saying in a fluting voice, "you're so strong, only you can stop Skeletor!"

Garret's seven year old daughter, in her best low voice, said, "Don't worry, She-Ra! I'll help you!"

Louis stopped playing, like an actor on a stage startled by the manager turning up the house lights. Looking around. Distracted.

There was a rumble you couldn't hear. Elena frowned.

Garret felt a kind of indefinable dread, coming out of

the very bottom of his gut in slow, diffuse waves of anxiety. Resonating with the unheard rumble in the air. A subsonic shiver.

Garret said, "You feel . . . anything? kind of like something's out of whack or . . . ?"

Elena hugged herself, and pursed her lips, and said, "No." Lying through her teeth. Looking up at her workroom window.

The rumble, again. Felt but not heard. Rising again—and then gone. Garret saw Louis shiver, and look around. Then Louis shrugged, and raised his She-Ra sword. "He-Man—Skeletor's coming!"

And Garret thought, for no reason in particular. *Contact.* It sounded in his mind twice, in the voice of some mental phone operator. *Contact.*

"Skeletor is here!" Louis said. "But so is She-Ra and He-Man!"

* * * * *

If you write poetry when you're a teenager, you probably write bad poetry. Especially if you were young in the late 70s, early 80s, with all the dour, gothic rock people around, and you were sensitive, a bit alienated, fairly smart. In that case, you wrote poetry that matched your clothes. Poetry dressed all in black, poetry with little silver skull ear-rings and kohl around its eyes and maybe a tattoo that said BORN TO DIE.

But bad poetry isn't meaningless. The day before Enter came, Garret was going through a box of press clippings in his office, looking for a nasty review of one of his own early bands—he was going to show it to one of the bands he was booking, to show them that arrogance was a perennial mistake. On top of a thin book of clippings, Garret found one of the high school notebooks he'd filled with bad poetry.

Found himself reading some stuff he wrote one night after his parents came home drunk—they always came home drunk, and usually left home drunk. Drunk and snarling at one another.

He was the child of alcoholics, with all the attendant low self esteem, fear of abandonment. The poetry, in consequence, could have been cited in a psychological casebook, with lines like:

Loneliness comes in concentric circles
Like the circles in Dante's Hell
And the innermost circle is the hardest to see.

Pretty heavy-handed stuff, he thought. Garish. But now, fifteen years later, it rang true, somehow. He was married, had two kids, once had a lot of girlfriends; still had a lot of friends. And he wasn't as lonely as it was when he was a young misfit teenager, no. But he was still a circle away from knowing anyone.

* * * * *

She came to Garret when he was trying not to masturbate. He was working late in his office, upstairs in their house. He had his feet up on the transparent plastic desk, next to the PC he never used, a cup of espresso in one hand—from the espresso machine on the file cabinet, a machine that he did use a great deal. He was making phone calls that simply seemed to breed more calls. He was trying to get the TinTones on the same bill with Wind Window, despite the irritating sound of the dual wordplay names, and at the same time fighting the randiness that had plagued him all week. He was tempted to slip into the upstairs bathroom, run through one of his repertoire of sexual fantasies, discharge some of the sexual tension. Then get back to work. But he knew it was a way to avoid sex with Elena. Sex they were overdue for. Something she was getting bitter and sarcastic about. So he was trying to hold the randiness in for her . . .

It happened when he was absentmindedly changing a light bulb. He was talking to Chalky, the Brit who was the manager of the TinTones, telling him, "I just talked to Bill Graham, and if you can make a concession on the band's paycheck—Hey, Chalky, man, this gig is an important showcase for the Bay Area because the programmers will all be there, especially the guys from KROQ and KNET—" The walls hummed with a distant, almost unfelt rumble. And then, *phht*, the overhead light burnt out, leaving Garret in a darkness broken up by streetlight glow coming bluewhite through the blue curtains. It was like suddenly being put into photonegative. But he kept talking to Chalky on the speakerphone as he got a bulb out of a desk drawer, stood on a chair, tilted the fixture aside, unscrewed the dead bulb. Telling Chalky, "You do this one for me, pal, I'll do one for you—"

And then a thick, shining, violet fluid dripped out of the empty light socket.

Pop. The sound of the dead light bulb breaking on the floor. Slipped from his fingers as he stared.

The glowing fluid dripped in slow motion.

As Chalky rattled on about something, "The trouble is, luv, I've got more people to please than just my dear, dear mate Buzz Garret. There's the promoter, the record companies . . ."

A filmy ribbon of purple and violet plasma was issuing from the socket, swirling and dripping, fluid but gaseous too; like smoke, but it wasn't smoke. It crackled softly and flexed itself like an idea. Unevenly lighting the room in twisty neon.

Garret said, numbly, "Chalky, call you back." Hit the

hangup button. Stared at the socket.

Some kind of electromagnetic peculiarity? Some kind of swamp gas sort of thing? A hallucination? Was he that stressed out?

The ribbon thickened and turned in the air, and took shape as it torqued, like a figure emerging on a slow lathe. The shape . . .

He thought of certain paintings by Georgia O'Keefe. And others by Judy Chicago. He thought of women.

The shape was mercurial and full of promise. It reached octopally toward him—

He fell off the chair, onto his ass. One hand went into a patch of broken light bulb glass, cutting the heel of his thumb. His butt hurt from the fall. He hardly noticed any of this. He couldn't take his eyes off the shine, the shape growing, getting big. Big as Mindy Gretch. Mindy, the ebullient expanse of nude Mindy Gretch, his first sexual partner. She was a two hundred pound nineteen year old glitter rocker, into Bowie and Alice and the Dolls. Davie Garret, at sixteen, was mesmerized by the Niagran fullness of her breasts. Mindy put on a chilling tough-rocker-chick act, and though the young David Garret identified with her outsider status, he was kind of unnerved when she asked him to come over to sneak some of her parents' vodka. Maybe she'd get drunk and kick him around or something. But that night in her parents' basement she was tender and tentative . . . Where was she now?

She was here, now. Standing there, nude, in his office. One of her eyes was smaller than the other; one of her breasts the size of an apple, the other enormous. She was listing to the side because one of her legs was six inches too short. Then the shape adjusted for parity, like a parade balloon inflating, and she was symmetrical. Her eyes and legs and bosoms equalized. The Venus of Willendorf with Mindy's face.

She was not quite there in the flesh. Her pink skin had a violet underglow, and there was a faint purple light in the very middle of her, shining like the filament in the new bulb he held in his right hand. The bulb, with no power source, for no damn good reason at all, was lit up in his hand. Glowing.

"Mindy?" She'd died, and this was her ghost. It was the only thing he could think of.

He ought to be scared. Instead he was disoriented and—

And drunk. It came over him like a wave of drunkenness, as if he'd had grain alcohol intravenously. A rubberiness, a pliancy, rippling through him. The room rippling with it too; a rumbling wave of The Unseen that passed through everything around them. It emanated from that purple glow at the center of her.

The drunkenness that was more than drunkenness kept him from screaming when she closed in around him.

Pop. The other light bulb hitting the floor, as Mindy clamped home around him like the jaws of a gentle beartrap. A great soft pink and violet trap.

He was surrounded by Mindys. Six of them, all interconnected somehow, seamlessly joined at the hips and rolls of fat at her middle; six Mindys facing inward, a circular accordion of Mindys, pressing against him, naked and reeking deliriously of flesh and female lubrication, six pairs of enormous Mindy breasts . . .

His hard-on hurt him.

The drunkenness left him inhumanly loose, but didn't leave him flaccid or numb or tired the way booze did. This was being drunk on Mindy.

She peeled his clothes from him. He had enough

rationality left to wonder what Elena would think if she came in, Would she even be able to see it? If Elena saw it would she scream?

Should I be screaming? he wondered, as he squirmed close to this Mindy apparition, felt her embrace on every part of him, all 'round. Closing in on him so he could barely breathe. Succulently warm.

Embraced by her at 360 degrees of the compass, the six interlocked Mindys around him, blended together at their hips and arms and legs; six faces, six pairs of breasts, six vaginas: six two-hundred-pound women symmetrically arrayed like fleshy petals, like the inner parts of a Claes Oldenberg flower, and for a moment he had a hideous, frightening vision of himself sucked into a venus flytrap made of this all-encompassing woman, sucked down into some sickening tube and slowly devoured . . .

But then she reached down, under her hugely pliable belly, and two of her hands guided his cock into one of her vaginas. Smoking with sensation as he entered her. Drunk with euphoria, a wallowing in woman . . .

Contact. *Hello.*

His erect cock was a phoneline to her, and the phoneline was open.

All lines are open, she said. *Call our 800 number . . .*

"What?" he asked. In a gasp, pumping into her. Into the purple shine at the mysterious heart of her.

Contact, she said, *You wanted contact.*

"Who . . . oh Christ . . ." Feeling like he could go on doing this forever. Standing here, making love to her. To all six of her. Hands exploring other orifices as his direct line to her jacked into the vagina directly in front of him . . . Six tongues, all from one woman, lapping at him . . .

"Who? Are . . ."

Identity. You're asking about my identity. She didn't say it, and she didn't exactly think it at him. She formed concepts and he became aware of them, but it was as if they were occurring to him with a kind of cognitive synchronicity he shared with her . . .

She answered his question, though he didn't know it for a while. She shifted. *Closer*, she said.

Picture a woman stretched like an image on silly putty, for one second; picture a strangely iridescent taffy in a transparent taffy-pulling machine, for about two seconds. Then the taffy loses its palpability, becomes a translucent matrix of light, for another incandescent second; then the light takes a shape in the air like an iris, a six petaled iris, each petal vaguely reminiscent of a woman, some undefined woman. The woman becoming less human but more palpable, more physical, as she flows over you . . .

This time it was an effort not to scream. But he was afraid that if he screamed, he'd disrupt the rapport, break some fragile balance between them, and he wanted desperately for what was happening to go on. The contact was an unspeakable relief.

So he didn't scream when she enfolded him like a cocoon.

His eyes were open, when the cocoon closed completely over him, and what he saw was something like the patterns in peacock feathers, but made out of the faces of women, women he'd known and women he'd never known, overlapping, sliding one into another. Faces limned in knowledge and perception; a depth of feeling he'd only glimpsed before. He thought of making love to them—his erection was as rigid as a radio tower, and it was transmitting-and the women's lips blossomed, sucking, nibbling, kissing; an organ that was both a mouth and a vagina drew his erection into it. His hands skied the curves of waists, the fullness of hips and thighs, the roundness of arms; every epidermal inch of him coming into contact with her: with them. With the tautness of skin over collarbone, the exquisite silk stretched under a jawbone, a sweetly slithering chain of damp labia drawn past his shoulder, down his torso; a padded room of buttocks and breasts embracing him; a glittering panoply of eyes looking piercingly into his. A bouquet of mouths sweeping past his genitals. Everything was wet but nothing was uncomfortably sticky; was redolent of flesh, sweat and lubricant, and all those scents and effluents melted together into a symmetrical harmony in keeping with the kaleidoscoping visuals of her. She was an endlessly reproduced variant on pattern, like the ornate embellishments of the Sun King's palace decor, but none of it was simple decoration; it was *expression*. And none of it was fragmentary; it was all of a piece, symphonically articulated by a guiding mind.

She was around him like a great vagina, his body the penetrating organ, but the organ that enclosed him was charged with radiant intelligence, and was at the same time the electric piquancy of all sexuality. He moved peristaltically within her, his entire body pumping through her. When he thrust out his tongue, a tongue arose to meet it. When he squirmed away from one vagina and thrust his cock in another direction, another opened to receive him. Breasts filled the hollows of his body. He swam between them. He could breathe, he could move freely, and yet she was everywhere.

He writhed to escape and at the same time yearned to stay within her. And light and flesh began to intermix.

Light and flesh were one, was all around him (somewhere, the office phone was ringing, ludicrously ringing again and again, answered by the answering machine, Chalky yammering after the beep, wanting to try some stupid scam on him,), sliding against him, interpenetrating his own skin on the waves of some exotic electromagnetic field, stimulating each of his nerve ends so that he was sweetly feeling everything, not with sensory overload but with sensory renewal. His erogenous zones beaming like kleig lights.

The boundaries began to dissolve. He was no longer able to sense clearly where his own flesh ended and hers began. A shattering panic whistled through him—and then was absorbed into a long slow undulation of reassurance from her.

You will not be destroyed in me.

He believed her. He let go. Felt himself turn head over heels. Saw himself from the outside . . .

And she shifted again. She was a specific someone, now. She was Jane Wasserstein. When was it? 1975? He was eighteen, she was seventeen, had jumped a grade. Jane, the girl he'd dated for five months before she'd broken down and . . .

And put out. What kind of expression was that, "put out?" It was both barbarically sexist and touchingly resonant of an adolescent boy's wistfulness. Put out: put it to the outside. Give, in a way that makes insiders of outsiders.

Here she was. Jane. Slender, curly blond, sylphlike Jane. A half-Jewish girl with asthma, who blinked rather often, as if her quick mind was taking in more frames per second than everyone else. Eyes like a blue-violet premonition of the underglow in this creature's skin . . . "Just don't say 'Me David you Jane,'" she'd said, on their first date, a breathless half second before he *would* have said it. Second date she'd said, "You going to ask me to go to the drive-in or are we going to work up to that?" She was always a step ahead of him. He felt like he was playing chess with her. He'd make a pass and she'd snort, "oh *listen* to him!"

The undefined woman had shifted, now, in 1989, in the office of Buzz Garret and Black Glass Productions. Mindy had become the shifting cocoon which had become Jane, Jane all 'round him, Siamese sextuplets formed in a circle, but somehow all variations of one, and not a confined joining of many.

He knew this creature wasn't Mindy or Jane. But drove himself into the nearest Jane, and made contact. Hello again.

Jane's voice, coming on as if triggered by a mnemonic answering machine. Something she'd said to him, when they were both seniors in high school. *David you're a professional misfit, and* you'll probably make big money at it like Alice Cooper or Frank Zappa. But you're not kidding me with this Rimbaud of rock act, all You really want is for everybody to love you, which is all every *Joe Normal wants too . . .*

No, he told her, that's not all. I want them to love me as I am. No matter how I am. I want that much acceptance.

Now, in '89, his tongue brushing Jane's small, hard breasts, her nipples becoming stiff as little .22 bullets, the electric contact of his tongue on her was like a switch triggering more astrally recorded memories.

Buzzard Garret, punk romantic. Jane's words, riding on a sneer, as she broke up with him in their freshman year at UCB. Two weeks before he dropped out to focus on rock. *You always had a* feel, David, for what women wanted to hear. They invariably thought it was endearing, too, that you were a punk romantic who could leave silver-spray-painted roses on a doorstep, quote morbidly romantic stuff from Verlaine in a letter, talk about psychic union in lovemaking, and still go out on stage and tell the world you hated it. That made you a tragic figure of romance, right? So why'd you do it, Buzz? Just to get laid? That was never enough. You insisted they had to fall in love with you. When I gave up the nookie, it wasn't enough. You had to make me say I loved you. You *fucking pig*.

She'd gone right to the heart of him. He saw himself, through this Contact, as she had seen him: He needed them to be in love with him. He needed them to believe he was in love with them. But he couldn't be, not really. He could say all the right things and make the right moves. Could give them a good semblance of sexual passion. Surprise them with romantic gestures, call them funny pet names. Could even marry them. But he could never really, honestly love them. This way, he had them under his thumb. This way he controlled them, and this way he was safe from abandonment.

And all the time he thought these things, he kept plunging into Jane. Who was not Jane anymore. She was Sandy. Pleasantly plump, busty, spray of freckles across her cleavage. The same exact pattern of freckles reproduced on six linked manifestations of Sandy all around him.

Because if you don't want to have a baby, Sandy'd said, *you're* not serious about living life. You're full of yourself and you'll *never live that way*.

She'd wanted kids, and he hadn't, and they'd broken up over it. After that he'd dated sometimes three women a week for three years, and then he'd met Elena while he was booking a college where she was working in the student affairs office, he was blown away by the crystalline vastness of her intellect, the subtlety and intensity, alternating, when she made love. Her odd combination of spiritual emphasis and hard science. *The Tao of Physics* ruling their lives. She'd got pregnant and informed him she didn't believe in abortions.

So okay, babies and marriage. Their conjugal lovemaking

was good up to a point till she realized he was holding back, holding back more than ever now that he felt trapped by marriage. Withdrawing more and more as the resentment in him quietly grew. Elena sensing it and withdrawing to protect herself.

Communication between them became businesslike or brittle with sarcasm and acrimony. They were caught up in the vicious circles of quietly angry marriage, endless reflections in a hall of mirrors—mirrors that were funhouse warped . . .

And suddenly, now, standing up in his office, he found himself making love to his wife.

Six of her, at first. Then, the six Elenas collapsed into one woman. Like a string of paper dolls folding up into one.

He was making love to an Elena with a violet underglow to her translucent skin, and a purple orb shining at the center of her.

He wanted to run. But then he looked into her face, and saw none of the sophisticated hostility that Elena normally kept there like a falcon in a cage. He saw only the basic Elena, perceptive, vulnerable, curious, private and more emotionally complex than he'd ever guessed.

The impulse to run faded. He sank into her, more deeply yet. His fingers tracing the hollow of her back, her buttocks, finding them entirely new; and finding that his hands were dipping into her skin, shallowly sliding through her skin as if it were a fur of electrically charged flesh.

And then he struck gold.

He drove deeper into her vagina, and the electrode of his organ made contact with the electrical receiver of hers, some inner node of sheer receptivity. Contact.

Hello.

"You're not Elena," he said, ludicrously trying to identify

her even as he feverishly pumped into her.

This time she spoke aloud. "Yes and no. Call me Enter. I need your help. I'm trapped in this otherness, trying to get to my husbandside. I'm trapped—" All the time both of them copulating deliriously, joyously, as she gasped into his ear: "Need your help getting through to the free level."

"What are you?"

"A consciousness; a body of different principles but similar essence. A woman. A connection to women, from your viewpoint."

"Where do you come from?"

"An otherness. Not this world; not this plane; not this universe. But with roots in it."

"How can I help?"

"Don't come."

"What?"

"You're about to have an orgasm. The electrical discharge that accompanies the reproductive discharge will come too soon. Don't come, David. Don't orgasm. Wait. Timing is crucial."

He saw it like a tidal wave on the horizon of his mind's eye. An orgasm rolling toward him with the inexorability of a force of nature.

He withdrew from her, just in time. The build of orgasm slowed, faded, stayed aching just on the brink of his groin . . .

He acted on intuition, or perhaps following some set of instruction she gave him through the secret connections they'd explored. He stepped *through* her, as if she were a door. Walked through Elena; through Enter, who became amorphous and plasmic. Feeling a shock that was almost a burn sear through him as he went. Coming out on the other side knowing that if he looked back, she wouldn't be there. But she *was* still here, unseeably, waiting for him to complete the favor.

He was standing nude in his office. Clothes heaped on the floor. Skin slippery with sweat and lubricant.

He walked to the door of his office, his erection wagging, transmitting, still, like a radio antenna. opened the door, the doorknob crackling with sparks under his touch. Walked down the hall to Elena's studio. The room she kept for her hobbies. The door opened for him, before he got there. No one near to open it.

He stepped through. Saw Elena lying back on the rug, naked, her clothes heaped untidily about her. She was panting, glistening with sweat. Her legs apart.

Between Garret and his wife was a low metal table. On it was an intricate design of copper and silvery metal, some sort of occult ideogram made of metals, wired to the electrical socket overhead. Shimmering with violet glow.

With some strange combination of quantum physics and ancient female witchcraft, his wife had invoked Enter, drawn her from another world, channeled her through this one. And drawn someone else too. He could feel his presence. The husbandside. The male one. The one Enter was trying to rejoin. He'd been here, making love to his wife, even as Enter had been making love to Garret.

Like Enter, he was gone now, from the visible world; but he was here.

The wave of intuition that had brought Garret to this room filled in the blanks for him: Elena had been desperate for contact. Found herself unable to break through to him directly. Blocked. Neither of them could bear the humiliation of a marriage counselor. So Elena had tried something exotic and indirect, a quirky synthesis of physics and ancient magic, never expecting it to work. Some personal ritual, performed for psychological reasons, which had translated into objective reality.

Don't question it, Garret thought.

He went to Elena, lay down beside her. The true Elena. He lay beside her and then with her, entering her very soon after the embrace began. Feeling the first orgasm buck through him. Breaking down the barrier between worlds. Enter passing through her to him; Enter's male counterpart passing through Garret to her. Enter and Husbandside meeting and joining and passing on, freed now, into their own world. Having left Elena and Garret transformed behind them.

Garret had a glimpse of something, just before Enter and Husbandside passed on. That Enter and her lover were one creature, with two aspects; two sides of one coin, meeting here where dimensions intersected. And they had connections, interfacings with other consciousnesses—with Garret's, and Elena's. With all others.

Garret made love to his wife several times that night. And each time—

Contact.

Thomas Roche first sent me bio info indicating extravagant sexual proclivities. Then he sent me a second more sedate bio with a listing of his extensive writing credits. Probably the only fair introduction is some amalgam of the two. Roche's work has appeared in a number of magazines including Black Sheets, Paramour, *and* The Ninth Wave, *as well as the anthologies* Splatterpunks 2, Dark Angels, Blood Muse, Ritual Sex, S/M Futures, *and* By Her Subdued. *Those last three anthologies featuring Roche's work should be available from Masquerade by the time you read this. He has also written for White Wolf's fiction anthologies based on* Vampire: The Masquerade, Mage, *and* Changeling. *Roche edited* Noirotica, *the brand new anthology of dark erotic crime stories also published by Masquerade Books. Sometimes he listens to way too much Lycia.*

Sticky Fingers

Thomas S. Roche

I was wearing the leather top that shows off my tits, so the private pig patrol didn't look too close at the backstage pass. It was the pass Roxy had forged for me on her computer. Not bad for such short notice. It wouldn't stand up to any serious scrutiny, so once I got back there I slid into the shadows behind the band equipment as I heard the security guards coming. I crouched low and tried not to move, knowing that if one of them caught sight of me I'd have to do it. But no one looked. They were too busy bragging about all the groupies they were going to fuck. Especially that aging porn star with the tit job. They'd heard she'd fuck anyone.

I had to fight to keep from busting out laughing. What a bunch of sleazebags. But I managed to hold still and not make a sound. I was a little cold in the shadows. It was a hot night, but then, I wasn't wearing much. My black stretch jeans were torn to shreds, barely hanging on — only a little of it from the pit at the concert. Underneath I had on garters and fishnets, which you could see through the holes in the jeans. I had cut the holes myself with my roommate's pinking shears. My boots were knee-high pointy-toed Goth boots with two dozen buckles. Didn't have much of a shirt, just this tight studded leather bustier Roxy had shoplifted for me from a leather shop once. It showed off the tat around my hips and the jeweled ring in my navel. I had a matching leather collar around my throat and of course I had all my piercings in.

Funny thing. Except for my facial piercings, I was dressed just like the chick in the last Deathtones video. I heard Lucrezia was really into her but she'd dumped her recently. Maybe it was a long shot.

The security guards were gone, and I slipped out of the shadows. I gasped as the cop surprised me from behind.

"What are you doing in here?" he shouted.

"Shit," I said, my heart pounding. "You fucking gave me a heart attack."

"What the fuck are you doing back here?"

He wasn't a real cop, just a security clone, in uniform. Jeans, leather jacket, and a NIN T-shirt. Long ratty hair halfway down his back, dyed black. A dozen silver earrings and a nostril piercing. Like I said — uniform. But I recognized him from the fan mags, and I knew who he was even if I couldn't remember his name. He wasn't a hired clone, he was part of Lucrezia's private security. Nobody important, but he'd have what I wanted. In more ways than one.

I smiled at him naively, then bit my lower lip, using my tongue to toy with the steel labrette, turning on my lust as hard as I could.

"I just sort of wandered back here. What's your name?"

"Never mind that, who the fuck are you?"

The guy's name tag said Robert: Security. Now that I wasn't so freaked out, I realized that he was pretty cute. Not like one of those big beer-belly scary motherfuckers. I could do it with this guy. If I had to. Maybe even if I didn't have to.

"My name's Trisha Rott," I said. "It's good to meet you, Robert. I write for Deathslutt magazine. I do that column, Waiting for the End of the World — you know, at the end. Back page, every month. Right after the poisonous recipes section. You know the publication?"

"I'm afraid not," he said skeptically.

"Yeah, I posed in it, too, last issue. You ought to check it out. I mean, I was in this girl-girl shoot — you know, with a strap-on. Real freaky stuff, with Maddy Cumm, you know, the porn star, all — well, anyway, you can probably guess. Course I had black hair then so you might not recognize me. I looked like this — " I struck a pose with my hips cocked just so, my hand curved around an imaginary and enormous hard-on like I was jerking myself off. I laughed, trying my best to seem stupid and horny, which I figure wasn't all that far from the truth except for the first part. I was trying to confuse the guy.

He reddened but looked sort of bored. "Right."

"Well, anyway, I just sort of wandered back here. They let me through. Is Lucrezia still around?"

"Let's see your press pass."

I took out the forged pass. Right there: Deathslutt. Correspondent. The two Ts at the end had been my idea. Never mind that the magazine didn't exist. The pig shook his head sadly, put the pass in the pocket of his jeans. "That's a sad forgery, Ms. Rott." He laughed. "Did you do it on a copier or something?"

"Call me Trish." I leaned closer to him.

He spoke slowly, calmly now, not taking the bait. "You're not supposed to be back here. Lucrezia told me she doesn't want anyone back here. Just security."

"You sure she wouldn't make an exception for me? She and I could to a girl-girl shoot, maybe with a strap on. . . though she probably wouldn't need one. Have you done her, Robert?" I was leaning real close to him now.

"Just forget about it," Rage said firmly. "You'd better turn around and walk out. I'd hate to have to. . . ."

"Strip search me?" I said blandly, getting impatient.

"Fuck off," he scowled, then seemed to think better of it. "Yeah," he said. "Strip search. I'd hate to do that. Look, this is getting old. Get out of here or I'll get you out."

"You'd have to touch me to do that," I said, finally pushing myself as close to him as I could get without touching him. "Then I could sue your ass or something. My dad's a lawyer in the City." I sighed sadly. "On the other hand, it looks like most of the other pigs are busy chasing their own tails, if you know what I mean. No reason to waste the window of opportunity." I toyed with the zipper on my leather top.

Rage was breathing hard. He made a grab for me, like he didn't know where to hold on. So he got me around the wrist and by the hair, turned me around and pushed me toward the exit, almost carrying me. I yelped as he pulled my hair and squeezed my wrist, it hurt like fuck. Then he pulled my head back and I went limp against him, which is exactly what he did not expect.

That's what I was planning on. It gave me just the room I needed to push my face up into his, hard, and get my lips against him. He was so fucking shocked that I had my tongue into his mouth and he was the one going limp — at least, his arms — while I rubbed my ass against him and felt the slick steel of his tongue-piercing sliding against mine. Excellent.

Then he seemed to get a new wave of resolve to show me the exit, and pushed me forward, dragging me hard.

I stayed limp, though, and next thing I knew I was behind the equipment, deep into the black shadows, and shoved against the brick wall. Rage was on me, kissing me hard from behind, grabbing my hair and pulling my head back roughly. He shoved his tongue deeper into my mouth and I pushed back, feeling the steel clack together as he Frenched me. He let my wrist go and I used it to reach back and feel his hard-on through his jeans. With my other hand,

I got the zipper of the leather bustier open. It fell away into the darkness, and Rage's hand closed over my tits. If he was surprised by the thick stainless-steel rings through the nipples, he didn't show it. I whimpered as he felt me up, and I kept groping at his prick.

He was a lot taller than me; he had to bend low to kiss me like that. So when I got his pants open and pulled him forward with my hand around his cock, he stopped kissing me and just looked down at me. He had great eyes.

He spread his fingers, squeezing my tits and tugging at the nipple-rings, which felt incredible. I kept staring into his eyes, my eyelids fluttering as he squeezed roughly — not too polite, this fucker. But he wasn't being overly careful with the piercings, just twisting and tugging at them, the way I liked, which made me squirm and rub my ass against him, smiling up and beckoning to him demoniacally with my tongue every time he pulled away from kissing me. Rage smiled back at me, pinching my nipple hard with his thumb and forefinger.

I arched my spine and pressed my tits more firmly into his grasp as he rubbed them and played with the rings. Rage pushed me harder against the wall. I pressed my buttocks against him and spread my legs, bending my knees and crouching down a little. He bent down to put his lips up close to mine again and gently teased my mouth with his tongue, letting me suck and nibble on it. Then, pressing his lips firmly to mine, he began to french-kiss me even deeper than before. I felt his tongue sinking hungrily into my mouth as he bit my lower lip hungrily. His tongue began to seethe into me. I felt his tongue parting my lips wider so he could thrust it deep into my mouth; I shoved back with my own tongue and felt Rage playing with it.

"You gonna do me?" I said, gasping when he pulled back for a second. I squirmed, pushing my ass against him.

"You know it," he said, getting my pants open wider so he could pull them down over my ass. I bent down and took my jeans and panties down to the tops of the patent-leather boots. While I was down there, I went to work on his pants with one hand and with my mouth while I did my boot-buckles with my other hand. It was his turn to lean up against the wall as I got onto my knees and pulled open his black jeans. His jockeys were soaked with sweat. I pulled them down over his balls and rubbed the head of his cock with my thumb while I put my lips against his shaft. He had a piercing through that, too, apadravya, well-placed. Careful not to suck on the head, where he was leaking luscious pre-come, I slid my tongue up and down and wrapped my lips around him. I used my tongue to get his balls into my mouth, sucking and kneading them gently. Then I was back up his shaft, smelling the inviting tang of his pre-come, that much hotter 'cause I knew I couldn't swallow any. That just made me want his cock more, just made me want him to shoot his load inside me. While I was sucking his prick I finally got all the buckles snapped on my deathrock boots and kicked one of them off so I could get out of my jeans and panties. Then I managed to get out of the boot other, and slipped off my jeans. Now I was naked. That's the way I liked it. I can't seem to fuck with any clothes on — call me a naturist. I like to be nude when I do it. Down on my knees still, I spotted the telltale bulge in Rage's jeans pocket and slipped one hand in each pocket, coming out with both hands full. Right hand: a Blackjack — my brand. With my left hand I palmed the laminated card from his pocket and got it slipped into the remains of my jeans there on the beer-soaked floor. He didn't notice, so I got back to work without missing a second. I tore the wrapper with my teeth, rolled the jet-black condom over his pierced cock and stood up, pressing against him.

"Time to earn that nickname," I told him. I turned around and leaned myself over the hard-plastic equipment crate, spreading my legs for him as I propped my upper body up on one elbow.

Rage came up behind me, guiding the head of his cock between my pierced lips. He pushed into me gently at first. I felt the thick latex-sheathed head entering me, and then he drove the shaft home. Rage slid deep into me and began to fuck me — hard, like I'd told him, like his name. He started giving it to me in deep thrusts, real hard, but real slow. It felt perfect. Pretty soon I was sprawled out on the crate gasping for air while he did me.

I didn't figure I'd get off — not in that position. I usually don't do it from fucking unless I'm on top. But for some reason the head of his cock kept punching my G-spot or something, so I felt this dull throbbing ache go through my whole body, pressing me closer and closer to a climax whether I wanted it or not. It felt so good I thought I was going to piss myself or something. Rage put his hands on my waist and held me down against the crate as he fucked me, grunting with each thrust. My hipbones were getting bruised but I didn't give a fuck. I just wanted him to keep fucking me. I urged him on, concentrating on getting closer to the orgasm deep inside my cunt.

"Oh god, yeah, keep doing it, just like that — just like that — oh fuck yeah!"

I came before he did. That seemed to surprise him a little, and I lost part of the orgasm as he stopped thrusting.

But I spat out "Don't stop now, asshole!" and so he kept thrusting, and before I was finished with my come his cock had pulsed inside me and filled the Blackjack with Rage's juice.

I just laid there for a moment, draped over the crate, as Rage pulled out, tied off the condom and tossed it into a corner.

When I felt like I could finally walk, I got up and leaned against the crate, watching him. Rage had a cigarette lit and was looking at me nervously. I began to pick up my clothes. My fucking underwear had landed in a pool of spilled beer and was soaked through. I tossed it into the same corner as the condom and put the jeans on without panties. I wiped my sticky fingers on the front of my jeans before zipping up the leather bustier.

Once I had my clothes back on, I asked Rage for a cigarette.

He handed me one and I lit it. Rage looked guilty.

"Look," he said. "Lucrezia's gone already," he said. "She took off right after the show. But I got a pass. . . ."

I sighed, rolled my eyes. "I know that. You think I'm a dumbfuck?" I held up the hotel pass I'd taken from his pocket. It was a hologram, impossible to duplicate or forge. Even for Roxy and her magic computer.

Rage laughed. "What makes you think I'll give that up? I'll call the hotel and tell them not to let you in. Tell them it's a bogus pass. Shit, I'll call the cops."

"No you won't. I'll tell them you sold it to me for a blowjob." I put the pass back in my pocket.

Now he was trying to bargain. "Look. . . .um. . . "

"Trish," I said.

"Yeah, that's it. Trish. Look, we can both go to the party. I'll take you as a guest."

I shook my head. "Be seen with you in public? That's not the deal," I told him. He wasn't that bad but I just wanted to twist the knife a little.

Rage sneered. "Seems to me," he said flatly, "we didn't have a deal."

"Exactly," I said. "That's your bad manners, not mine. Next time sell what you got, OK? Everyone'll be happier."

I left him there red-faced and walked toward the back exit. I knew Roxy was out front waiting for me in the car.

I've been in love with Will Judy's writing ever since I first discovered it at a party at his mother's house in Potomac, Maryland, when I was seventeen and drunk. Apparently alcohol doesn't dull my aesthetics any. Today, Judy is the copy editor for Blue Blood *and a frequent contributor to both* Blue Blood *and the* BLT *humor zine.* Blue Blood *is currently serializing "The Mercy Agenda", Judy's noir novel of cult intrigue and bisexual sub/dom entanglements. Will Judy used to break strings in various DC area bands, but he claims to hate all musicians, particularly bass players. Go figure. On the other hand, he loves mean women, coffee, Raymond Chandler, and his grandfather's old gun in no particular order. The fucker also managed to crash my hard drive when modeming me the final edits on this story from some den of iniquity in Seattle, but don't hold that against the story. I'm trying not to.*

Temporary Assignment
by Will Judy

In my head I can hear perfect music, but only sometimes. The first time I was five, at the dentist. A big day : first cavities (three of them; I couldn't stand the taste of toothpaste), first drugs (sweet nitrous oxide from a nose mask), and the first sour taste of the drill. It bored into my head with a spectacular flash of blue that leapt like a gas flame, and the noise that whined through my jaw to my ears dropped and modulated with each wintry pull of gas until it was low shimmering drone that rolled under me like a highway. And the wind that channeled through the dry bones of my skull finally blew me into the arctic, all pure white ringing light.

The last time I heard the music in its full bloom was with you, when you broke my nose for me. I am a stupid, stupid boy. My reasons for needing to remember you are as pointless to explain as the reasons for any of the other things I do.

As pointless as giving up on school again, after one more frictionless semester of browbeating teaching assistants in discussion sections and scrawling obscenities during lectures. This particular bout I had been showing up for classes and handing in papers with some regularity, so my grades had even been good. And one day, sitting in some cafe trying to kill a headache by swilling coffee, watching text run off the pages of a ravaged library book, I realized that I had spent over an hour fantasizing about beating everyone around me to death with my bare hands, and perhaps a chair. I needed out, again. I canceled my summer classes and broke the news to mom and then dad, who could not even rouse themselves to anger anymore. Then I called my agencies, who did not remember me.

Summer is the worst season for temping. Everyone is out of school, and kids wanting beach money for August will take jobs at half the standard rate. Turn down too many assignments and you get shitlisted. Knowing this, I did not turn down the warehouse job when the phone rang at 7am.

It was not a promising assignment. July's latest heatwave was pounding the roof like a kettledrum; it was too hot for coffee. The agency had sent five of us, and we all had the same haunted look, standing at the bottom of another canyon wall of boxes stacked on skids. And then there was you, with your clipboard and your cutoffs, perched on the front of a loader explaining our mission. None of us listened to a word. We didn't have to. After a while you pick it up by contact, which isn't as flatly insulting as actually listening to the way people address you - like kindergarten teachers, talking through you, not hearing anything but short, simple answers. If you thought we were paying attention, it was likely because we couldn't stop watching.

They were all looking at your purple hair and probably thinking that freaky girls will do anything in bed. I was looking at your purple hair and thinking that you hadn't stripped it before dyeing it, and that you weren't likely all that freaky, just a plain girl with straight brown hair and no makeup, on vacation from a good college, pissing off your folks by doing prole work. You looked happy, though unsmiling, pleased to be standing there in your black t-shirt and eight-hole Docs telling a bunch of grunts to put what where. I watched you, not listening, and I liked a few things about you. I liked the strong, trim line from your shoulders to your thighs; swim team muscles, I imagined. I liked the way you absently swiped away the hair that stuck to your forehead with the side of your hand, like a cat grooming its ears. And I especially liked the darkness under your eyes, the only color on your smooth white face. Insomniacs always have a certain cachet of sleep about them, a morning puffiness like clean sheets just slept in.

I didn't much care for anything else about you. I especially did not care for the ease with which you kept yourself above us, always finding something to stand on as you scratched at your clipboard or called out orders, never addressing any of us directly. And I didn't like you being younger than me and there for the summer, I didn't like your fading dye job, I didn't like your unpierced ears, I didn't like having my uncharitable notions confirmed when you showed up one day in your cutoff college T-shirt. In a perverse sort of way I liked that you went to a women's college, because that added the possibility that you were a four-year dyke as well.

Not that I gave a shit. My co-workers all wore headphones, so I had no one to talk to, and all I could do all day was haul boxes and think. If I thought about you, it's because you were there and more interesting than a cardboard box. And every once in a while, if a real workflow was established, a solid and thoughtless rhythm, I could listen to the ghost music in my head and forget about you.

The job dragged out longer than expected, which suited me. August is the last crap month of the season, and September meant all the students and public school teachers would go back to their little burrows and clear out the office jobs. September would be air conditioning and ergonomic chairs, and now I didn't have to worry about the August bills. The delay had you pissed off, of course, since you were our supervisor and it reflected badly on you that things weren't getting done. By Thursday of the last week, you were starting to show some loose ends, which suited me as well. It was stinking hot, and all of us were slowing down badly enough by mid-morning that you let your clipboard drop to your thigh and told us to break for lunch early, addressing some spot on the ground about four feet wide of where we were working. I was the last to stop work, as usual, and when I swung my box up onto the skid I caught your eye by accident and saw a flash of real anger that made me snap my head away. I tried to walk away from it, but I was tired and dehydrated and not really up for a quick reverse, and I wound up stumbling and sitting down fast on a lucky box. This left me sitting on my hands and haunches like a rabbit with you looking down at me like a coyote. This seemed to amuse you, which made me mad. I fixed you in my sights and took a deep breath.

I don't think you listened to a thing I said, actually, but I'm sure you got most of my points just from tone. I wasn't listening to you, either. We were both just standing there boiling in the soggy air, gusting at each other. I don't remember getting up and I don't remember you climbing down from your perch. I do remember a sudden break in the noise during which I was the only one shouting, like when the music cuts off in a club and you're the only one singing, then a feeling like a puff of wind and a huge pressure in my sinuses. I got my hands up in time to catch a long splash of blood spilling from my nose, and my memory replayed the sight of you throwing a long open-handed slap at my face. The fact that it only takes six ounces of pressure to break someone's nose from the side was obviously never drilled into you.

We were both immediately all business, no disbelief or apologies, just Shit, get me to the can, I can't see, and All right, hold my arm, this way. We banged through a door or two and I felt myself jammed up against a sink and heard you twist the tap. I leaned down and scooped water to rinse my face. Opening my mouth wide and raising my eyebrows, I got my eyes to pop open. I saw you in the mirror standing behind me, looking genuinely interested in what I was doing. With the blood watered down, my nose didn't look that bad, just slightly displaced.

"Doesn't that hurt?" you asked.

"No. It's like having a really bad stuffy nose. Setting it might be nasty."

"Okay. I'll drive you to the hospital. Do you want to..."

"No, you don't have to."

"No, come on. Let's get going."

"No, look, it's not that bad, and anyway I don't have insurance."

That stopped you for second. I'm sure you were going to say something about workman's comp, and it struck you that fighting with your supervisor wasn't covered.

"You don't mean you're going to leave it like that.."

"No."

Silence.

"Maybe you don't want to watch this..." I said.

"Bullshit. You aren't going to . . ." And our eyes met. Yours were dark chocolate brown, almost black because your pupils were so wide. I placed two fingertips on either side of the bridge of my nose. Instead of looking at the mirror I looked at you.

"No fucking way," you said, smiling for the first time.

I smiled back, and snapped my nose back into joint with an audible crunch. I did not quite faint. When the pain released me I realized that I had fallen forward and you had

caught me, both of us tumbling back against th
closet-sized employee pisser. We were forehea
giggling stupidly.

"How many times have you done that befoit
asked.

"Never." And I had to kiss you.

I remember so little. But I remember it so well.

You met my kiss hard enough that I had to step back
and catch myself on the sink. My hands shook for a moment,
then steadied against your hips and began a slow glide over
the cool sheen of sweat on your back. I could not breathe,
and gasped as that first kiss broke, then growled as you sank
your teeth into my straining throat. My fingers bunched
into your sweaty shirt, and you straightened your arms and
stepped back out of it, revealing heavy breasts mashed into
a jogbra.

I had a moment of deep adrenal terror when you
fumbled behind you for the doorknob, followed by a wave
of coolness when I heard the lock click.

You hooked your thumbs under the shoulder straps,
stretching them and peeling down. I watched, amazed at
how lush you were and how you kept so much body so well
disguised. Then you sauntered up and draped your strong
arms around my shoulders and let your chest flatten warmly
against my spattered shirt. I dragged my fingertips up your
ribcage and kissed you as I palmed the sides of your breasts,
pressing them together. You bit my lip when I experimentally
pinched your stiffened nipples. Your hands moved to the back
of my head; you pulled me down and I bit your collarbone.
You pulled harder and I bent my knees, dipping my head to
kiss your tits, tickling your nipples with my circling tongue.
You dug your nails into my scalp.

I came up for air and you sank your hand down the front of my jeans, collaring my burgeoning cock with your cool fingers; your shoulder working as you tugged at me. I eased your cutoffs down over your round, muscled ass, stroking your hips; you went up on your toes when my fingers found your fever-warm cunt.

You levered down my jeans and rubbed your clit with my cock-head, the thrill of all that heat and wetness arched my back and bristled my neck. You smirked up at me, and without breaking eye contact for an instant, slithered down my body until my cock bloomed from the sweaty hollow between your breasts. You bent your head and I whimpered softly as you brushed the crown with your lips. You looked up, took in the look on my face with pride, and extended your tongue to stroke me languorously from base to tip. You took me in by degrees until I could feel your breath on my belly, then pulled back effortfully, your cheeks hollowing, your lips softly sputtering.

You were showing off. I did not mind. You glanced up at me occasionally as you made your slow, torturous progress back and forth; considering and calculating.

When my legs began to quiver, you disengaged. You kissed my hipbone, stood, steadied yourself with a hand on my chest, and kicked your shorts from around your ankles. I kissed your face and turned you so I could hug you from behind, then ran my palms down over your breasts and belly to your thighs, and then back up. My left hand cupped your breast, my right forefinger traced its way along your inner thigh to the humid flesh of your cunt.

I gripped the back of your neck in my teeth, took a nipple between my thumb and forefinger, and stroked you from back to front, starting at your perineum and settling into a long spiral around the hard knot of your clitoris. You arched against me, stretching like a cat, and ground your tensed ass into the underside of my cock. I nibbled along your neck and circled your clit, slowing to match the grinding of your hips and shoulders. Your head lolled back, and I kissed your face; when our lips met, you pushed away from me and turned.

You faced me for a moment, then stepped forward. With your arms around my shoulders, you boosted yourself up on to me and hooked your legs around mine. I got a jolt of pain as my fumbling hands were caught in the hot collision of our coupling.

Your voice was close in my ear, supervising as usual, and then saying nothing at all. I came first, and my helpless bucking brought you along with me, your slick thighs clamping around my hips.

And I remember the two of us crumpled on the floor, muscles slack and cool, and the echo of the careening blue roar of perfect guitars in my ears.

We helped each other up, groomed each other as well as we could. A few paper towels and you looked better than before; my shirt was bloody and my eyes were starting to blacken. Getting out inconspicuously turned out to be disappointingly easy, as no one was back from lunch. I had to get home and tape up my face, so we went and got my bag and you walked me to the loading dock, confusedly fussing with me . I stumbled along, dazed, telling you not to worry. When we rounded the corner I wanted to kiss you again and found that somehow I could not. I touched your cheek and looked to meet your eyes, looking in them for something I could not name then. I do not remember saying good-bye. I do remember looking back once to see you standing up on the loading dock, high above me once again, arms folded, a slight breeze moving the ends of your hair.

I wore sunglasses driving home, and managed to do a fair job on my nose with some micropore tape I had appropriated from a hospital job earlier in the year. I spent the rest of the day in my room, ringing away at my guitar. When I went in on Friday to take care of my time sheet, you were not there.

The air-conditioning of September came and chilled my bones, and my nose healed without incident, itching like hell while the bone knitted, but leaving only the slightest bump. And when the first leaves began to turn, it became clear to me what I was looking for in your eyes that day.

There is a vast difference between a Temp and a dilettante, the test being whether or not you have something to go back to. More simply: Whether or not you have a choice. You left and went back to your scholarly room and some braying Film Major, or, for all I know, some shouldery woman from the crew team in your bed. Next summer, you'll be building houses in Nicaragua, after that you'll be a Summer intern at some oversized magazine in New York. Then graduation, a wander-year on the continent, a job and the conveyor belt to the cemetery. You could have been summering in the Hamptons for all the difference August will make in the course of your life. But you chose this.

I don't have a choice. I have no intelligent explanation for why I can't hold a proper job or finish a degree, except that after any real length of time in the same place, doing the same thing, the music I can catch snatches of every once in a while stops cold. My life has to stay fragmented or I can feel myself start to die. I will very likely live my whole life this way, wandering, running, touching nothing truly familiar. Knowing this creates a desperate need to leave something behind.

I don't care what it is you remember. You do not know me at all. You do not know of my travels and failures; my fear of water or my passion for Dashiell Hammett. You do not know that I found unimagined reserves of strength to keep my shaking legs under me as you ground yourself against me. You do not know that I hear perfect music in my head. Sometimes. If the face that I saw in your eyes is all that stays with you, I cannot complain. A small, permanent position.

Cecilia Tan founded her publishing house Circlet Press in order to encourage eroticism in science fiction. Circlet titles have included Worlds of Women, Blood Kiss, Feline Fetishes, TechnoSex *and a collection of Tan's own short fiction called* Telepaths Don't Need Safewords. *Her work has also been anthologized in* Noirotica, Looking for Mr. Preston, On a Bed of Rice: An Asian American Erotic Feast, By Her Subdued, *and* Herotica 3 *and* 4. *Tan's versatile writing can also be found in a number of magazines including* Blue Blood, Penthouse, Paramour, *and* Sandmutopia Guardian. S/M Visions, *Cecilia Tan's anthology of erotic science fiction, should be out from Masquerade by the time you read this.*

Rock Steady

by Cecilia Tan

I'd been playing bass with Sardonyx two months when I started to lust after Alan. OK, no, you're right, that's a lie. I lusted after him the very first time I saw the band play live, at the Shake-n-Bake (what a dive), when they opened for Glimmer Twitch. Sadie, my ex-girlfriend, was "singing" for Glimmer at the time (more like howling and peeling off her clothes from time to time), and she'd begged me to come to the show. Not sure why, but she put me on the highly touted guest list (which at Shake-n-Bake means you only pay $2 instead of the regular $5 cover, whoopie), so what he fuck, I went, I hung round back stage, and when Sardonyx went on stage, I went out to see them out of sheer boredom.

They were hot. At the time they were all men. Alan thrashed his guitar and sang like a wild man, sometimes into the microphone, sometimes not. His coppery blond hair was just long enough to cover his eyes. Short, stocky Midge sat behind the drum kit like he was some kind of kick drum himself, steady and solid. Then there was the bass player, an asshole named George. Chill out, girl, I thought when I found myself clapping and hollering between songs. But I wanted more, more, they were so hot, so tight, it was the kind of rock I liked with a heavy move in the bass line and buzzsaw guitar. Call me a post-punk purist.

When they came off the stage I had walked up to Alan and told him I thought it was a good show. He'd tossed me one of those condescending looks, you know, like I was a groupie but not fuckable material. Well, fuck you, too, is what I was thinking, but deep in the pit of my stomach I still wanted him between my legs. I put it out of my mind.

Two weeks later Sadie called to say that George had gotten so pissed drunk (again) at a gig that they'd tossed him out of the group and were looking for someone new. OK, fine, I thought, I'll audition, I'll see His High-and-Mightiness again, what the fuck. It'll probably just be the waste of an evening, but it wasn't like I had a lot else to do. I still had four months of unemployment coming to me after the layoff and couldn't spend every waking hour job hunting, could I? (Regardless of what I had to make the unemployment office believe...)

And bang, I got the gig. Alan didn't seem to remember me at all, just had some vague notion I was a friend of a friend of someone's and so he should be nice to me. We dove into rehearsals and getting me up to speed since Sardonyx had a pretty full schedule that summer.

Two months later, though, it started to get serious. We were doing a show at Randy's Lounge (don't laugh, it's a cheesy name but it's actually one of the coolest places to play) and there was this electric tension in the room. We were rocking and I had almost forgotten to be nervous. See, I'd been in a couple of bands here and there, but never really played out very much, and suddenly I'm doing four or five shows a month and I'm petrified the other guys will figure out I'm not a "real" musician. Anyway, picture this: I'm laying down the beat, thick and heavy with Midge pumping the kick drum, and I slowly wake up to the realization that I'm humping the bass with every note, my thighs are humming, and I'm wet. And there's Alan, creeping toward me as he solos, grinding his hips while the notes soar...

At the time the thought I had was: maybe I need to get laid more than I need a job. Well, I suppose I'm in the right line of work for getting laid, eh? Well, not exactly. When the set was over and the gear was packed, Alan and Midge had their pick of groupies—I wouldn't have minded taking one of those sweet chickadees home, myself. Even Carl, Midge's cousin and our official "roadie" got hit on. But I got nothing much but a couple of leers from the unshaven, beer-bellied sound man. And it struck me (not for the first time) that there are some things that are cosmically unfair about being female.

That night I had a dream. There we were, on the stage, the same pumping rhythm throbbing in the background, and Alan was taking one step after another toward me. Suddenly I was naked except for my bass (a burnt-cherry Rickenbacker and one of the few things I blew a couple of paychecks on back when I was employed in the real world), and lying on my back on the top of an amp, the thud coming from it making the throbbing in my clit stronger. Alan's pointing his guitar toward me now, and the head slides in up to the nut... wait, I think, is that a guitar or his anatomy? And who named them that, anyway?... but it doesn't matter, in the dream, something is sliding up my cunt, filling me up, and it feels so good, so good. My hands keep playing, thump, thump, thump, but my legs are spread wide for him and I never want it to end.

Of course, I wake up, though, the dream dissolves, and I end up jamming my fingers into my panties and trying to picture someone else, Keanu Reeves, Winona Ryder, anybody other than Alan, but my brain keeps looping back to him and I think: shit, this is serious.

Because you know all the twisted shit that can happen when people in the same band start sleeping together. It's like when housemates start doing it, or coworkers, or maybe it's the most like incest (I can't speak from personal experience on that one), where the people involved have all kinds of messy interconnections and there's more at stake than STD's. It's okay when people who are already sleeping together start a band (Wings? Well, maybe that's not a great example) or move in together (that's called marriage). But when you're already in a band... it's the whole shitting where you sleep thing, I guess.

Two days later at rehearsal, I got to hear all about Midge and Alan's masculine exploits. Whenever we took a break, we'd sit out on the concrete loading dock of the building where our cinderblock-and-acoustic-foam practice space was, and smoke and yack. They'd gotten used to me being around and didn't try to couch their language or anything anymore. In the beginning Midge'd say "fuck" and then he'd apologize to me, or Alan would trail off before finishing a sentence. Maybe that one time I'd grabbed my head and whined "ooohh! My virgin eeeears!" they got the hint that they did not have to excuse their French. Even to Carl now I was just like one of the guys. So now I got to listen to every technicolor detail of their amorous adventures. Oh man, I thought, wouldn't it just be the greatest if I did bag one of those groupies, take her home and rock her world? But well, I probably still wouldn't be crude enough to tell these guys about it, shock value or no. It was one of the reasons Sadie had dumped me—she claimed I was too repressed, didn't know how to relax around sex. And well, I'd countered, maybe if I ever got some I'd get used to it. That had shut her up. Sadie could be mighty frigid when she wasn't too depressed to feel anything at all.

Anyway. Much as the thought of taking home a groupie was entertaining, there was still the gnawing attraction I had for Alan. Okay, maybe Sadie was partly right, since there's a fine line between repressed and suppressed. I decided the wisest course was to shut off the hormones and ignore my libido. I had enough things to worry about, didn't I? We were working on a new tune Midge had written and he wanted to do this very funky rhythm section thing. Now, while we worked out the parts, I felt Alan's eyes on me. I will not flub this, I will not flub this... But I still hadn't nailed the part by the end of the night and I went home feeling rather empty. I thought about calling Sadie—hearing about how fucked up her own life was often cheered me right up—but the twisted way her mind worked she'd probably be in bed with Alan before the week was out. Instead I lay on my futon in the dark, staring at the stripes from the blinds on the ceiling and running my fingers over the fretboard of the Rickenbacker.

You're kidding yourself you can keep this gig, I thought. You could save yourself a lot of trouble if you went back to job hunting, quit the band, and then you could fuck Alan's brains out with a clear conscience. But despite the seeming logic in that conclusion, I knew it wouldn't work out so neatly. I mean, if I quit Sardonyx, Alan'd probably never want to speak to me again, much less sleep with me. And then what? Well, I guess I'd have even more time for job-hunting. It all seemed pretty pointless no matter how I looked at it.

But you know, the subconscious doesn't stop rolling because the rest of the brain got its knickers in a twist. I fell asleep and had another one of those dreams. In this one, I'm in a very dark, enclosed space and there's this kind of constant low-level hum... my mind starts weaving explanations—this is a tour bus I'm sleeping in—and suddenly I'm huddled next to somebody. My brain conveniently fills in Alan. He's pressed against me and his breath is warm as his fingers dig through the covers and clothes to slide across my stomach.

Two fingers are pushing their way down into my panties, down between the folds of my slit, down into the crease that became instantly wet as soon as I felt where those fingers were going. He slips them inside me and begins fucking me like that, all the while his mouth near my ear, the dark closeness of the space all around, I'm suffocating deliciously in sensation. This is what dreams are like.

The next morning I think to myself: that's two heavy penetration dreams in a row. Maybe I should buy myself a dildo. No wait, I remind myself that I've decided to forget about sex and I push it to the back of my mind.

If I were an accountant or a chef or a postal worker (or a clerical worker, which is what I was before the layoff) this plan might have worked. Ignore your lust and the waiter/mail carrier/cute guy in the next cubicle you have the hots for will eventually fade to the background. But in rock and roll, everything you do is sex. Every song you sing is about sex (or death, or both), every move you make is sex. The words "rock and roll" even mean, literally, in the old slang they came from, "sex." So this lust I had for Alan was sort of always there, and the dreams came pretty often for the next month or so.

Toward the end of the summer Warren, our sleazoid booking agent, set up a bunch of dates for us to play some bars and rock clubs in upstate New York. Midge, being a drummer with a lot of shit to lug around, had a van, so we three piled into it with all our gear and took off for Syracuse. Or was it Albany? Van like that, two people sit up front and one in the back. I lay down in the back and slept most of the way where we were going to that first gig.

Let me tell you something about booking agents. They don't give a fuck. They aren't the ones who have to put up with their great planning jobs ('oh come on, it isn't that far to Rochester' 'yeah, from Canada!'), their money saving ideas ('it's good weather for camping'), or their lameness when dealing with club managers. Warren had set us up in a bunch of college towns while school was out of session and the club owners hadn't lifted a finger to promote the shows. That first night we played for twenty people and then slept at a campground where the running water wasn't running. Midge had brought a little dome tent, barely big enough for two, then insisted that Alan and I sleep in it. He wanted to spend the night in the van, paranoid that it and/or our gear might get ripped off by grizzly bears hungry to start a power trio. Alan just shrugged and crawled into the tent. I crawled in after him and pretended to go to sleep. Lying there next to him, I couldn't quite get comfortable... okay, that's an understatement. We were both sweaty from the show, the ground was lumpy and uneven under me, the round tent was the wrong shape for anyone to sleep in much less the gangly length of Alan and he had curled into a ball leaving me a crescent moon-shaped sliver to lie in. So I lay there for a long time, breathing in the sweet scent of his sweat, curled around him but trying really, really hard not to touch him. In my mind, I played fantasies that only made it worse: he was faking it too, and would suddenly roll over and confess his own suppressed lust for my gorgeous body, or, he would wake up from an erotic dream and, too horny to go back to sleep, would beg me to help him... It was another one of those cosmically unfair situations. Playing a show, even a kind of lame one like that night, is always like a kind of foreplay. It gets the juices pumping. Does anybody really not get that connection? Famous rock stars don't fuck only because pussy gets thrown at them. They're primed for it. So, end result?

I spent most of the night wallowing in a pool of hormones and frustration. Weird thing is, the next day, I swear he got friendlier. More familiar. Putting his hand on my shoulder, shit like that. And on stage, he seemed to spend more time in my orbit, playing back against back, sharing my mike.

Not that the ten people who showed up to see us cared all that much. The club refused to pay us. I talked Midge into letting us rotate who slept in the van and he and Alan took the tent. After the third show, where there was a sizeable (okay, 35 people) but openly hostile crowd, we got paid $50, and the owner tried to claim that our mike stands and cords were his, Midge and I were all for packing it in, canceling the other three dates, and going home where we could sleep in our own beds, have hot showers, things like that. But Alan wouldn't hear of it. "Oh, come ON," he said. "Why did we bother to come out here? This is good for us." Apparently the adulation of even a minuscule number of people was enough for Alan. I was surprised a little by this fact. Camping out hadn't made for any groupie liaisons and I'd thought the lack of nookie would have made him more cranky than any of us. But he rallied us to persevere. The next date was Ithaca.

We arrived to find the bar where we were scheduled to play closed. Not closed permanently, just "Closed Wednesdays" as the sign on the door read.

"Is it Wednesday?" Alan said, standing there with his hands on his hips. "Is it fucking Wednesday?"

"It is," I assured him, "Wednesday."

"This is just fucking great." He kicked the door with an unsatisfying thump. "Now what?"

Midge folded his arms. "I say we find a liquor store, go to a motel with hot running water, and get rip-roaring drunk."

It seemed like the rock and roll thing to do. I suggested one modification to the plan once we were back in the van— that we find and pay for the motel first before we spent all our money on booze. In the end we had about thirty dollars we could blow and still have money for gas. We stocked up on hard cider, Pete's Wicked, Southern Comfort, and Mad Dog.

You can guess what happened next, right? I mean, I wouldn't have bothered to go through all this build up if there wasn't some pay off, yes? We got drunk first, of course, which is everyone's excuse for the fuck they might regret or want to pretend to forget. Alan and I on one bed, Midge on the other, we drank and watched cable TV, Alan flipping between MTV and a slick, high-budget porn movie where hairless-pussied starlets were being fucked in a fountain. Sometimes it was hard to tell which channel was which. I was fascinated by the porn, though. I hadn't actually slept with a man for two years or so and I'd forgotten what a naked, erect penis looked like.

At one point I realized Alan was looking at me.

"What?"

He gave a little smirk. "You're so... into this. Your eyes are bugging out of your head."

I probably blushed but I tried not to. "Give me a break," I said. "Not everyone's such a pervert that this stuff is commonplace." My eyes returned to the screen where yet another erection was being revealed in all its glory as another actor doffed his briefs. And straight men watch this? I thought to myself. Amazing. "So tell me," I said, "why do guys always lie about their penis size?"

Alan snorted. "Guys don't always lie. Sometimes they exaggerate."

"Okay, but when they say 'eight inches' where do they measure from?"

Midge laughed.

Alan thought about it for a moment. "Well, from the base."

"Yeah, but what do you mean by base? Is that on top of it? Or do they inflate the figures by counting from the balls or what? It's still a lie."

"You know," Alan said seriously, "I don't think there's been a lot of development of a scientific method of dick measure."

"Well, where do YOU measure from?" I was definitely drunk or I'd never have said anything like that. Would I?

Alan scooted close to the TV and pointed with his finger to the actor humping on the screen. His finger moved back and forth and the guy's hips thrust back and forth with almost blurring speed. "See, from here."

"No. There's too much movement."

Alan frowned. "Look, it isn't that hard to figure out. If you really want to get technical about it, every guy should have to give more than one number. Length from the top, length from the base of the balls...."

"Don't forget width," I said. "How about total volume?"

"Yeah, whatever. I mean, I'm six inches measuring from the top, which is like nine inches from the underside, you know? So I could just say 'nine inches' and not qualify that and who's going to know? That's what guys do."

"No way are you nine inches," I said.

"Yes I am."

"No, you're not," I challenged. "You're just lying like all the rest of them."

He stood up. "Okay, all right. I'm sick of women

making male-bashing statements like 'guys always lie about their dick size.'" And he began unzipping his jeans. I didn't think he'd really do it, but he showed no signs of stopping. I felt like I should say something to stop him, but I didn't really want him to stop.

Midge snickered but didn't say anything.

Alan pushed down his briefs to reveal a beautiful erection. I don't know how else to describe it. Neatly circumcised, his cock curved upward at a graceful angle and had a certain symmetry about it. The sight of it made my mouth water and my loins ache. I thought about all the dreams, where his fingers, his guitar, or unseen appendages were fucking me in the dark. Now I could see the tool for the job and I wanted it.

"See?" he said. He measured off the length on the top with his fingers. "On top, this long. On the bottom..." he reached between his legs, "this long." And held his hands up for comparison.

Midge eyed him critically. "Well, that's not quite nine inches."

"But it's close. This isn't an accurate measurement, asshole."

All right, I'd had enough. I'd tortured myself long enough. And I was drunk enough. I reached a hand toward the shaft pointing toward me and gripped it gently in my fingers. It felt sweet hard, rigid but velvety, and I tugged him closer to me. "Mind if I borrow it for a while?"

Alan was staring down at me now like I was a total stranger. Which, in a way, I suppose I was. His gaze flickered from my face to his cock sheathed in my hand. Then he turned to look at Midge.

Midge got up. "Three's a crowd," he said, and went

out into the hallway.

As soon as the door closed, Alan took my hand off his cock and pushed me slowly but firmly back onto the bed. He climbed on top of me, his cock pressing hard against my pubis, and said. "Okay, you want me? I only do it one way."

"What do you mean?"

"I mean, I only do it like this. You lie where you are and let me do the shopping. That's the way I like it, that's the way we're going to play it, okay?"

"Okay," I said, not sure why he was so particular about this. But what the hey, I'd had lovers who liked to pretend they were dogs while they fucked. This was no big deal.

He started by stripping off my clothes. When I tried to help he held me still with one hand and pulled at the clothes with the other until I gave up and let him strip me. Then he lifted my knees and spread my thighs wide.

"Oh, Sandra, you've got a nice, dripping pussy here." He ran his hands down my thighs but did not touch my cunt. I thrust my hips up a little at him, wanting to feel what his fingers would really feel like down there, but he tsked and let my legs drop. "First things first." He lay down the length of me, still wearing his t-shirt, and kissed me on the lips. After a few tentative kisses, he let his tongue out and explored around the inside of my mouth. After a few minutes of that, while he continued french kissing me, one of his hands strayed to my breasts.

I figured it out. It reminded me uncannily of my first real sexual experience with a boy when I was sixteen, on a school ski trip. I had lain there while he undressed me and did all the work, starting at "first base" and working his way along until eventually he had his fingers up my cunt. At that point I dared to touch his penis and he had come, which dampened his spirit of exploration and we had stopped there and never spoke to one another again. I wondered if Alan had started out with this pattern, too, and just never deviated from it? He was so earnest about it, this routine. I imagined him using it on groupie after groupie... it probably worked like a charm.

He fondled my breasts for a long time, first with one hand, then he stopped kissing me and used two hands while he looked lovingly at what he was holding. He kneaded them like soft dough and then flicked his thumbs over my nipples until they hardened and I gasped. "Ah, that's good," he murmured as he began to suck on the hard buds. While he sucked, his fingers began to stray again, this time to my cunt.

I spread my legs for him and he stroked back and forth with the palm of his hand, dragging it over my clit and labia, the whole pubic area. I suppose that way he figured he couldn't miss. And he began to talk more. "Oh yeah, baby, nice and wet for me, nice and hot for me." He narrowed his hand to one finger sawing at my slit, then crooked the end of it into my hole. He ran his finger around in a circle and I moaned. "You want my cock, don't you."

"Yes."

He got up on his knees but kept fingering me. "Look at me. Look at it."

As I do believe I mentioned, it was easy to worship this cock. It was redder now, and I wanted to touch it, to lick it, to help me get ready for having it inside me. But his eyes told me to stay down.

His finger made deeper circles. "You're tight, so tight, Sandra. Are you sure you can take this?"

I didn't know if that was a rhetorical question or a real one so I stayed still and didn't answer.

"You sure you want this?"

Okay, that was a real one. "Yes."

"All of it?"

"Yes."

"All six-or-nine inches of it?"

Quit paraphrasing Robert Plant and put it in me, I thought. "Yes."

He pulled his finger out and smeared the cock head with my vaginal fluid. Then he got off the bed for a moment and I thought: oh, how thoughtful. He was putting on a condom. One less thing for me to worry about.

He returned to kneeling between my legs. If anything, his cock looked bigger now that he'd manipulated the rubber into place. He pressed the head against my cunt and rubbed it back and forth there, over my clit, smearing my juices around. Then he sank in about a half an inch. "Okay, Sandra, convince me."

"What?"

"I said, convince me. This is what I say to every girl I fuck. I don't go any farther than this until I hear it from you that you want me to. That you are absolutely sure you want to go through with this. That there is no doubt it your mind that you do not want me to stop right now and forget about the whole thing."

I put a hand on his chest and stroked him, marveling at how he could hold himself up like that. Was it just that I was drunk, or was he kind of twisted? He'd wanted me to lie there and not even move while he had his way with me, until now, when he was insisting he wouldn't go any farther unless I convinced him to. "Is this some kind of anti-date-rape strategy?" I asked.

His voice returned to normal for a moment. "Exactly.

You think I don't worry about whether some chick I pick up at a show is going to try to hit me with a lawsuit in the morning? I ain't giving her STDs, my sperm, or an excuse to complain." Now his arms started to shake a little and he dropped back into his husky seducer voice. "So if you want it, now's your chance."

"I want it."

"But do you really want it? Or are you just horny?"

"I really want it."

"You want this long pole of man meat inside you?"

"Yes!"

"Deep inside, grinding around, sliding in and out, pinning you to the bed, no mercy until I'm satisfied?"

"Yes! Yes!" I tried to pull him down onto me. He held off for a second, but I wrapped my legs around him and pulled myself another inch onto him. He let his weight drop then and as I sank back into the mattress he sank into me. True to his word, he began to grind. It was a tight fit, but I didn't mind.

"Oh, Sandra," he said. "I never imagined you had such a hot little cunt. Oh, I would have been fucking you since day one if I knew you were this good."

I didn't answer that.

"Yeah, mmm. I always thought you were a dyke, because of Sadie, you know? Are you a dyke? Did I convert you?"

I pursed my lips. "No, you didn't convert me. I slept with men before. Just not...." I sucked in my breath as he doubled his speed. "Not in a long time."

He pressed my knees up toward my chest and began slicking in and out fast, slapping our bodies together on the springy bed. "Oh yeah, you like that don't you."

My voice was kind of quavery as I said "As a matter of

fact, I do. If you keep it up, I'll probably even come from it."

"Oh, baby, you'll come. Don't worry, you'll come."

He was right about that. I didn't even have to sneak a hand down to twiddle my clit. The angle and the rhythm and the speed and the duration all worked together such that some time later, after we were both completely soaked in sweat and I began to wonder if he really could keep it up long enough... I began to scream. I mean really screech. But the orgasm had been building for so long, and my breathing had gotten so hard, screaming just seemed like the natural thing to do. And somewhere in the midst of all the noise I was making, he came, too.

I blanked out for a while then, blissed out, laying there in a wet, happy heap. I forgot who we were, where we were. It wasn't until he got up to throw the condom away and said "I wonder where Midge got to?" that I remembered—oh shit, I just slept with a bandmate.

Alan seemed to remember it, too. He came back and sat down. "This isn't going to turn into a psychodrama, is it?"

"I hope not." We eyed each other, wary now.

"You gotta make a choice, Sandra," he told me. "Now you've had a taste of it. You gotta decide if you are going to be a cock worshipper or if you're going to be on the other side."

"What do you mean?"

"I mean, you're either a groupie or you're on the stage. Can't be both. If you're a groupie, I can't respect you any more, can't work with you any more."

You are really twisted, I thought, but what he was saying kind of made some sense. "You mean, after tonight, you'll still respect me in the morning?"

"Hell yeah," he said. "After all, we're both drunk."

"Right," I said. "Okay. Where are we playing tomorrow?

Rochester? We better get some sleep, bud. That's a long drive."

He nodded. He climbed into the other bed (Midge never did come back—he'd fallen asleep in the van) and that was the end of that. I didn't have any more dreams about him, he never propositioned me, and Midge never mentioned it. I still don't get laid anywhere near as often as they do, but what the fuck, it's a living.

I first met Nancy A. Collins when Blue Blood *spokesmodel Sarah Mckinley Oakes and I went to go see her speak and ended up flirting with the sexy sixteen-year-old son of her husband the ever-charming Joe Christ. (Unless, of course, Joe lied to me about the fatherhood thing in order to watch me squirm.) Later on, Collins contributed "Demon Lover" to* Blue Blood #2 *and another short story to* Blue Blood #6. *This past summer, White Wolf released* Midnight Blue, *an omnibus edition of Collins' Sonja Blue vampire novels including one previously unpublished. The Sonja Blue cycle is by turns humorous and ultraviolent and enticingly sexy. Her werewolf novel* Wild Blood *has a similar feel to it. Her short stories have appeared in numerous anthologies including* Phobias, Confederacy of the Dead, Shudder Again, The Horror Show, Best of Pulphouse, Thrillers, After the Darkness, Splatterpunks, Hotter Blood *and others. Collins has also scripted such comics as* Swamp Thing *for DC Comics and* Jason vs. Leatherface *for Topps and acted the part of a quadriplegic who gets sexually assaulted for her filmmaker husband. She's done it all.*

Demon Lover

by Nancy A. Collins

Sina couldn't squat in front of the television set and act as if nothing was wrong between the two of them any longer, so she decided to go out and catch some live music, shrugging off Mike's silent reproach as he watched her from his spot on the couch. She knew she'd have to deal with his pouting when she came home, but she didn't care. She had to get out of that house or go mad.

When she pulled into the club's parking lot, she saw a man loitering in front of the building. He stood with his hands in his pockets, one leg drawn up, the boot heel resting against the door frame. He was cool and he knew it. The wall behind him bristled with staples like a buzz-cut porcupine. The bar's door was open, allowing the music to thump and crash its way onto the street.

As she drew closer, she could see he was tall and lean, with a finely muscled waist. His hair was blond and cut so it fell across his brow with practiced nonchalance. His eyes were electric blue, cold as witchfire. They were the eyes of a white tiger on the prowl. Something detonated in her the moment their eyes met. She grabbed a quick breath in order to steady herself. Excitement turned the oxygen in her lungs into ice crystals and helium. A blond. Funny, she'd never been attracted to blonds before. She normally preferred dark men, the closer to the Mephistophelean ideal the better.

Her throat constricted into a dry tube and her ears filled with the sound of blood. She felt clumsy and ridiculous, but there would be no running away. A horrible giddiness surged through her, just like the time she'd taken nitrous oxide at the dentist prior to losing three wisdom teeth.

Sina hesitated, digging into her pocketbook for the cover charge. She could feel the stranger's gaze flicker over her like lasers. She looked up, forcing herself to keep from trembling. He was studying her, his lips compressed into a flat, unreadable smile. His eyes were those of a debased angel, blue as Depression glass.

She quickly looked away and moved into the thundering dark of the club. She didn't have to turn to see if he was following her. She could feel his presence, as if joined to him by an invisible cord.

The club was close and smoky, the walls painted flat black in an attempt to create the illusion of space. The band was thrashing away on the stage, surrounded by a knot of wildly flailing dancers. She winded her way to the bar and was startled to see him already lounging there. The only open space was at his elbow. Setting her jaw, Sina moved next to him and ordered a beer.

She had to fight to keep from gasping aloud when he shifted his stance, his hip rubbing against her like a friendly tomcat. The beer bottle shook as she lifted it to her lips. The sexual arousal she was experiencing was so powerful it was almost unpleasant. Her crotch ached just looking at him. But what could she do about it? She wasn't drunk enough to simply swagger up and tell him to take her home and make her like it. She'd been out of circulation too long. She'd forgotten the anxiety and paranoia inherent in the mating ritual. What if he didn't want her? What if he was gay? The stainless steel death's head leering at her from his earlobe didn't help matters, either. As much as she loathed frustration, she feared rejection even more.

"I noticed you were looking. See anything you like?"

For a moment, she didn't realize he was actually speaking

to her. She blinked rapidly, as if startled from a daze. His face was inches from hers and she inhaled his musk, pleasantly redolent of masculine sweat. Her brain froze like a rabbit pinned by the headlights of an oncoming car.

He's bad news. You can tell by looking at him. No. On second thought, don't look at him. Don't do it. Don't say anything. Finish your beer and go home.

All attempts at witty remarks, sly come-ons, and last-minute escape fled. Her prepared speech died in her throat. All she could do was answer with the truth.

"Everything."

His name was Feral. He smiled when he said it. He pulled her onto the dance floor, hi personality sinking its fingers into her will. Every time he touched her she felt her skin tighten, as if mild electric current had passed between them. She'd forgotten the exhilaration that comes with a sensual high. When Feral wearied of dancing he suggested they go outside. The night breeze rapidly cooled the sweat on her body, making her shiver.

As she leaned her back against the wall, Feral tucked his left leg between her thighs and ground himself against her hips. It was an incredibly juvenile, but deeply gratifying public display.

He kissed her, his tongue probing with expert thrusts. His arms encircled her, locking around the small of her back. She felt like she was in a vise and, for a few brief moments, he lifted her on tiptoe. She could not control her breathing or pulse. Her fingertips vibrated against his skin.

Feral disengaged himself from their embrace and motioned for her to follow. He ducked into the alley that flanked the club, negotiating the garbage-strewn passageway with the grace of a panther. Sina wasn't quite as certain and hesitated, letting her hand drop from his grip. Feral turned, and it seemed for a moment as if his eyes were actually glowing in the darkness. Then he reached out, quick as a snake, and drew her to him, capturing her left wrist and pinning her arm behind her. There was no violence, no struggle, just the sound of their mouths meshing. Feral's free hand explored her body under her blouse, his fingers tracing the curve of her ribcage, squeezing her nipples and rubbing them with the ball of his thumb. She gasped and writhed against him like a cat in heat. His mouth covered hers and she had to remind herself to breathe.

Feral backed her up against the wall, plucking at the snaps on her jeans. His erection, coiled in his pants, looked like a hibernating snake. Feral reached down to pull on his belt buckle, and for the first time since she'd followed him onto the dance floor, she spoke.

"No."

Sina freed her left arm and placed her hand atop his own. Feral stopped, his blue eyes questioning her. What could she say? That she was scared of fucking him? He'd think she was some kind of neurotic cocktease . . .

"No, Feral. Not here. Not like this." She nodded to the heaps of reeking garbage that decorated the alley. "I deserve something better than this."

He stood there for a second, weighing what she had said, then nodded. His hand dipped into his jeans pocket and came out with a motel key.

"When you're ready, just come on over. I'll be there."

* * * * *

Sina sat on the edge of the bed and stared at the man she'd once imagined she would spend the rest of her life with. She knew she should feel guilty there was so little remorse to be scavenged from the death of their five-year-old relationship, but the guilt refused to show.

She studied Mike's familiar features, now rendered alien by the hollowness inside her. She tried to remember what it had been like, before the tedium and resentment leeched the passion from their lives. Her head began to throb. She closed her eyes, trying to summon pleasant memories of their life together. The years she and Mike had spent together had not been *perfect*, but they had been free of the pain and anxiety that been so much a part of her life before then. At first she didn't mind the long evenings at home; after the numerous chaotic affairs she'd suffered through, it was somewhat novel *not* to party every weekend.

But there had been problems from the very first. There was no way she could overlook that. Although her previous lovers had proved to be highly unstable, and treated her like shit, sex with them had been like walking on live coals and swimming in the Arctic Ocean at the same time. She'd found it dismaying that sex with Mike lacked the frictions she's grown accustomed to. She'd nursed the hope that as they grew together as a couple, their sex drives would eventually adapt accordingly; his increasing while hers decelerated, until they reached a suitable, mutually satisfying compromise. Unfortunately this never came about.

At the end of their first two years together, Sina marveled over how they'd succeeded at reaching a level of stagnation it had taken her parents two decades to attain. She began to experience an ill-defined postcoital dissatisfaction. She no longer made advances toward Mike, preferring to accommodate him whenever he felt the urge, which thankfully proved to be infrequent. Sex, once her drug of choice, had become housework.

Part of her chastised herself for being silly. So what if sex with Mike didn't sparkle? He cared for her, in his way, and respected her. He offered her shelter and stability. She forced herself to recall her earlier relationships; the ones that had left her -- emotionally bruised and physically battered -- on his doorstep in the first place. The memories were sordid, tinged with self-disgust and more than a little excitement. The dissatisfaction grew.

After their fourth anniversary passed without comment or celebration, she finally admitted that she'd been deluding herself all along. She'd never truly loved Mike. She'd simply needed a safe harbor to recover from the mistreatment she'd suffered at the hands of her previous lovers, and she'd mistaken his stodginess for stability. At first she'd felt guilty for being unable to transcend the demands of the flesh, but that was soon replace by resentment for Mike's inability to provide her with what she needed. He could not save her from herself and she hated him for that.

It was sheer accident she'd come across the poem.

When she read of the nameless woman, wailing for her demon lover, her face burned with the heat of recognition.

She realized she was mourning the lover she'd gone so long without. The demon lover she'd pursued in all his varied, imperfect guises for nearly a decade. For in order to taste the love the poets rhapsodized about, you have to suffer. To love as the immortals do is to know damnation. And the closest she'd been able to come had been the self-destructive, cruel, vampiric, parasitic relationships she'd found herself in with Jerry, Alec, Christian, Matt, and the others whose names, faces, and genitalia had now blurred together in her memory. They were men incapable of love, yet capable of inspiring suicide threats.

The longing continued to grow. She couldn't close her

eyes without seeing disembodied sex organs pumping away like Victorian steam engines, but she was hesitant about taking action. She still remembered Lee and how he'd dislocated her shoulder and blackened both her eyes. She had loved him with a passion that was close to maniacal. She'd lost control that time -- and it nearly cost her her life. And it had certainly robbed her of her self-respect.

One evening when Mike was not home, she went out to a bar, intent on screwing the first man who looked at her sideways. Once she got there, she discovered, she couldn't settle for just *any* man.

The older men in their synthetic fiber suits were ridiculous, if not actively repellant. Sina visualized them naked: paunches overshadowing their erections, their bandy legs white and absurdly hairy compared to their heads. The younger boys in their acid-washed jeans and silk tour jackets didn't fare any better either. They were incapable of appreciating the lyricism of sexuality; all they were interested in was hopping on, getting off, and pulling out.

She'd left alone, returning to her and Mike's apartment by herself. But it was not from a desire to remain faithful. There's been no demon lover there to satisfy her. She knew when she finally found him the recognition would be immediate. Her heart, soul, and womb would know him the minute she saw him. And tonight she'd finally found him.

Feral was the one she hungered for. She glanced at Mike's slumbering form, his back to her. She'd promised herself to sleep on it before acting on Feral's offer, and she meant to keep that promise. She climbed into bed next to Mike, pulling her limbs tight against her body in order to keep from accidentally touching him in her sleep.

She needed to get her head straight and think about

what had happened. She had security, a home, and someone who cared for her. She couldn't throw that away. Could she?

When she closed her eyes Feral was there, shimmering like an ice sculpture in the Mojave, and she knew what her decision would be.

* * * * *

The motel was every bit as seedy as she'd expected it to be. Men like Feral didn't shack up at the Hilton. The motor court centered around a swimming pool with fungus-dappled tiles and a basin spider-webbed by slippage. An overweight woman in maid's whites pushed a housekeeper's trolley along the second story promenade. It was hard to tell if the towels on the cart were clean or dirty.

Sina stood outside the door to Feral's room, working the key between her fingers like a rosary. She was walking the razor's edge. She'd almost forgotten what an exquisitely scary experience it was; like hanging over an ice chasm with nothing but a piton for support.

I should leave now. While I can. I could still go back. Mike would never know the difference. We could start all over again. I could do it. She unlocked the door and stepped into Feral's room.

With the curtains pulled and the lights off, the room was as dark as a movie theatre. There was a stake, closed odor permeating the air. Something heavy struck the carpet, as if someone had fallen from the bed onto the floor.

Feral's voice came from the darkness, his tone urgent; "Close the door! Now!"

Sina did as she was told. Here eyes had grown accustomed to the gloom, although she found the smell stifling. Feral was visible from the chest up, watching her intently as he crouched behind the double bed, his elbows propped against the mattress. She wondered if he was a pusher. If so, she was lucky she didn't have a bullet in her head for walking in unannounced.

"Feral . . . remember me? You gave me your key . . .?" She took a hesitant step forward.

"Sssina." The way he rolled her name around in his mouth sounded strangely sibilant. "Yes, I remember. I've been waiting for you." He pulled himself upright, exposing bare white flesh down to his waist. He appeared to be supporting his entire body on his forearms, the muscles as pale and rigid as marble. Sina was relieved to find the insides of his arms free of needle tracks.

His chest was hairless. In fact, except for the champagne-colored hair on his head and his slightly darker eyebrows, Feral's entire body was as smooth as glass. At least, those parts of his body she could see. She took another step toward him. Funny, he didn't seem to have either nipples or a navel . . .

Feral smiled and moved to meet her, gliding from behind the bed. His naked flesh glowed in the near-dark, as translucent as opal. His penis and testicles were overlarge and as she watched they grew to full erection. It was almost enough to take her mind off the fact that, from the crotch down, Feral was a snake.

He was at least fifteen feet long, from his pointed ears to the tip of his tail, legs merging into a seamless column as thick as his torso. Like his human upper-body, Feral's serpent half was as pale as milk. Sina was reminded of the albino snakes found in deep caverns.

Feral moved like a cobra, holding his human-self upright as he slithered forward. He towered over her, swaying slightly with every ripple of his abdomen. The revelation of Feral's inhumanity was nowhere near as terrible as Sina's realization that she still wanted him.

Feral's erection was now parallel with her sternum, his amber hair brushing the mottled plaster ceiling. His eyes were still blue, only now the pupil had become reptilian. She could not look away and she recalled how, as a child, her grandmother once told her about snakes charming birds out of trees and into their jaws.

"I've been searching for you for so long." Feral's voice managed to sound earnest, despite the forked tongue. "It took me so long to find you . . . to pinpoint the source of the Call that drew me from my place in Hell . . . I'm sorry I kept you waiting all this time . . . I can only move amongst your kind at night . . . I was afraid I'd never find you . . . But your Call was so strong . . . so persistent . . . it would not let me rest until I found you."

Feral swayed forward slightly, struggling to keep his balance, causing the head of his penis to brush against Sina's chin. It felt velvety smooth and pleasant against her skin. To her own surprise, Sina kissed the exposed glans, already glistening with a drop of pre-ejaculate fluid. Feral hissed in pleasure as she took him into her mouth, his cat-slit eyes rolled back under a nictitating inner eyelid.

After a few deft strokes of her tongue, Feral made a choked cry and pulled himself from her mouth. He swiftly wrapped her in a moon-pale coil, his scales whispering against her flesh. Funny, he didn't feel slimy at all. He felt so good she wanted his touch all over her body. She fumbled at the buttons and snaps of her own clothes, her fingers made clumsy with lust and gasped as his scales brushed against her naked flesh. Her hands caressed him and Feral hissed his pleasure. What was left of her sanity fled as she felt herself respond to his sinuous constrictions and undulations.

Feral's coils tightened, lifting her upward. She clasped his forearms, and as she reached up to kiss him, Feral's split tongue flickered out tasting her moans. Sina pressed herself against his cool, dry skin and shivered as his powerful fingers expertly tweaked her nipples. For the first time in her life, she was truly happy, cradled in the coils of a demon who'd braved the dangers of the mortal world in search of his human lover. She wrapped her legs around his waist, lowering herself onto his erect penis with a sob of pleasure. She gave another, sharper cry as his second penis emerged from its hiding place, penetrating her anus. Feral moved against her with a boneless grace, fucking her with a strength, agility, and depth impossible for a human male. Sina cried out at as the first orgasms took her, throwing back her head and giving voice to her pleasure like a madwoman.

* * * * *

"So, this is it, huh?" grinned the john. He smelled of Southern Comfort and his words came out slurred. He wore an ill-fitting polyester suit that did little to hide the beer belly hanging over his belt. He stuck his hand up her skirt as Sina unlocked the motel room door. "I bet you bring all the guys you pick up here, you little slut."

"That's right. All of them."

She opened the door, motioning for him to follow. As the john crossed the threshold, he sniffed and made a face.

"Phew! It sure does smell in here! You need to air this place out!"

"Don't worry. In a little while you won't notice at all," she assured him.

The john giggled and licked his lips. "Ain't that the truth."

As Sina locked the door, Feral moved from his hiding

place in the bathroom. The john had time for one muffled shout before the coil silenced him.

After making sure the prey was suffocated, Feral and Sina quickly stripped it of its clothes and wallet. The naked john's belly overshadowed his pubis and his legs were hairier than his head.

Sina tossed the wrinkled polyester suit onto the mound of similar objects in the corner of the motel room. She'd have to make another trip to the Salvation Army pretty soon. She retired to the bed, leaving Feral to finish what he'd begun. She'd gotten used to the sound of cracking bones, but she still had a hard time watching when it came time for him to unhinge the jaw. However, he wasn't the only boyfriend she'd had whose table manners left a lot to be desired.

She stuffed the bills and travelers' checks into the shoebox she kept stuffed under the bed and dumped the credit cards and other ID into a paper bag, to be disposed of in the nearest dumpster.

It wouldn't be much longer before someone noticed what was going on. But by then they would be well on their way home. At least Feral's home. He made it sound really nice, not at all what she'd been lead to expect. She was looking forward to meeting his folks, even though the prospect made her a tad nervous. After all, every girl wants to make a good impression on her future in-laws.

When I first met William Spencer-Hale, he was working as traffic manager at White Wolf and writing a bunch of stuff for their Gothic punk roleplaying games Vampire: The Masquerade and Werewolf: The Apocalypse. "Music of My Damnation" first appeared in Blue Blood #3. Hale left White Wolf a while ago to concentrate on his own writing and create Quintessential Mercy Studios. Hale's company publishes Luminary, the gaming mag for adults and is expected to come out with the Rapture roleplaying game some time this year. And, yes, Rapture is about what it sounds like. In his spare time, Hale hangs out at various Goth fetish clubs around Atlanta, Georgia and at various hotel bars around the country, where he lets really hot women fight over him. Hey, everyone needs a hobby. And, if you saw his woman, you'd probably fantasize about what she would look like covered in oil in a boxing ring with . . . uh, never mind.

Music of My Damnation

by William Spencer-Hale

The throb of the techno-beat pierced his brain like an ice pick. Darwyn sat quietly at the darkened bar, holding the scotch and water that he had ordered nearly an hour ago away from his body as if it were a severed head. He glanced apathetically over his shoulder to view the pitiful mortals thrashing about in time to the music, each attempting to dance more seductively than their peers. How he hated their pathetic little mating ritual. Every male attempting to be so cool and erotic as they throw their bodies around to the beat, every female so coy and mysterious behind her dyed-black hair and thick eye liner. It was the same ritual every night, perhaps the faces changed, perhaps not. They all looked so much alike it was hard to tell. He wondered if they could even identify themselves in this darkened cavern of sweat and pheromones.

Darwyn sat in silence as the fog machines belched forth their cotton-candy aroma and began to obscure him from the other patrons of the club. He had always liked it this way; being virtually alone even in a crowd. He could peer through the haze and watch the shadows dance wildly about the fog, seeming to have no source of origin. It was now that he felt the most comfortable. Still, he could not allow himself to feel at ease. Mortals could not be trusted.

Darwyn wondered, as he often did, who was the more cursed of the two species? The vampire, like himself, cast into a life of stark loneliness, forever driven by the lust for warm blood or the humans who constantly pretend to be something more than they are in their futile quest to find love and companionship. At least Darwyn had accepted his loneliness, it was a lesson that most humans had yet to learn.

Darwyn stood up, smoothed over the wrinkles in his black leather trench coat and carelessly brushed his long chestnut-hued hair from his eyes. As a passing thought, he extinguished the cigarette which he had lit some moments ago but had not bothered to smoke. It was time to go. He glided across the dance floor toward the exit. The mock-goth patrons of the bar made way for him as he did so, creating a tunnel of sorts which led to the escape of the cool night air. Humans could always smell a predator. As the fire red glow of the exit sign illuminated his face, he caught a reflection in the corner of his mirror shades, a reflection that, for a moment, almost made his dead heart beat again.

He turned to look, not believing that someone so beautiful could possibly exist, let alone be standing so close. But Darwyn was wrong. Before him stood something more than human, even more than vampire. A vision so lovely that it shamed him for being the monster that he was. Darwyn stood motionless, speechless as her eyes met her own in the reflection of his mirrorshades, although seeming frantic to find his. He slowly reached his hand up to remove his glasses. Apprehension began to creep into every fiber of his being as he feared that her image was nothing more than his own subconscious reflected onto the surface of his glasses. Once more, Darwyn was wrong.

She was still there, her long, curly, fire-red hair falling softly upon her shoulders as she fixed her eyes into his. Darwyn felt himself gasp as he peered deep into those dark green orbs. He watched as they mutated the reflection of the gathered crowd into something akin to dancing angels. Angels which danced to the music of his damnation. He peered deeper still and was lost.

Darwyn felt a soft caress on his right hand and it served as the means of travelling back from whatever dream world he had been transported to. He looked down to view it's source and spied his vision once more, smiling nervously up at him. It would seem that this was real.

"Who are you?" Darwyn managed to stammer over the migraine inducing blur of techno-noise. "Please . . . have we met before?

"Yes!" She replied with a gasp, her eyes holding frantically onto Darwyn's. "We must have, you seem so familiar." She stood as if frozen, her fingers gently caressing the curves of his palm and thrilling in the icy tingles that it sent up her arm.

"You're so . . . cold. Why?"

"I'm dead." Darwyn replied matter-of-factly, expecting her to flee from him and his dream to suddenly end as so many had before. Instead, she simply smiled and gazed away, her expression reminiscent of one remembering a dream.

"What is your name?" Darwyn asked, surprised that she still stood before him.

"Dance with me." was the only reply that she gave, her eyes once more locked onto his as she tightened the grip on his hand.

She exerted just enough force to guide him away from the crowded exit and back onto the dance floor. Once there she cast away her inhibitions and threw herself into his waiting arms. Darwyn closed his eyes and smiled to himself although he silently wept for her in the darkness of his heart for she knew not what the night had in store. As one they danced, grinding their bodies together in time with the music, eyes locked as they each searched for answers to questions yet to be asked.

The bass throb of the music grew faster in intensity and

so did their passion. Darwyn smiled to himself once again as he felt her hand slide up the length of his thigh and come to rest upon his cock. He reached around, cradling the warm flesh of her ass in his hands, pressing her closer to him as he did so in order to feel her breasts, soft and warm against his chest. His mouth found hers, their tongues fighting for dominance over the other as they glorified in the taste of one another. Darwyn felt his erection growing larger with each passing moment and so did the mortal angel that cupped it in her hand. She stroked the length of it beneath his torn denims in time to the music, frustration beginning to play across her face because of her inability to grasp it fully.

Darwyn pulled back and broke the lock that their lips had made. He gazed down upon her without a word and her silence was all the answer that he would require. He took her by the hand and led her toward the exit, passion boiling within him and guiding his every step. She followed closely, not wanting to lose her lover in the confusion of the crowd. Within seconds they were outside, yet the cool night air washing over them did nothing to extinguish the fires of their lust.

Once in Darwyn's midnight blue Carmen Ghia, they rumbled out of the parking lot toward the heart of the city and Darwyn's apartment. It was only seconds before her desire overpowered her once again. As Darwyn drove through the crumbling expanse of the city, his new-found partner slid over and began to slowly unbutton his jeans, a coy smile etched upon her face as she did so. She reached in and removed his cock, still throbbing with passion as it had back at the bar and began to slowly stroke it once again. She smiled to herself as she looked up to see his expression. Darwyn's eyes were half-closed and his lips were slightly parted as his lust overcame him. Without wasting any more time she softly kissed the head of his cock and then opened her mouth to accept it. Darwyn sighed aloud as he felt her hot tongue run up the underside of his cock. She was pleased with his reaction. She began to slowly glide her mouth up and down the length of his cock, each time stopping to lick the pre-cum from its swollen head. As she did this, Darwyn reached around her and cupped her breasts through her blouse, kneading each one in turn as she lovingly sucked on his erection. She suddenly stopped but only long enough to remove her blouse and bra in order to easily facilitate her lover's desires. Once this was completed she immediately thrust her head back into his lap and filled her mouth with his cock.

Darwyn began to drive faster, wishing that he did not live so far away from the club and as he accelerated, so did she. She was no longer holding back in her lusts, her intentions were quite clear. She had reached around behind herself, lifted her skirt and moved her panties aside, her fingers rubbing her swollen clit with the same attention that she gave to the throbbing cock that filled her mouth. Upon viewing this, Darwyn knew that he could not hold out much longer and gave himself completely to his lust. She seemed to sense this and she tried to take more of his hot meat into her mouth with every stroke.

* * * * *

The car suddenly stopped as they arrived at his apartment, but she did not falter in her passion. She would have her reward. She continued her pace as before, intoxicating herself on his musky scent as she lightly scraped her teeth across his cock each time that she came up. Unable to stand it any longer, Darwyn grunted as the semen began to build;

he had reached the boiling point and could not turn back. He grunted as his cum erupted into her mouth. As he came, so did she, her screams of pleasure muffled by the spurting dick that she held tightly in her mouth.

Their tide of passion subsided, but only for a moment. They exited the car, still half-dressed and rushed toward Darwyn's apartment. Once inside, Darwyn wasted no time and pressed his lover against the wall. She responded by tilting her ass outwards and spreading her legs wider. She looked over her shoulder to see her lover looming over her, preparing to enter the folds of her warm cunt. Their eyes met once more and he could sense her pleading for him to hurry.

As he entered her, he felt the walls of her cunt contract in orgasm. She screamed, this time unimpeded in her cries of passion and her sighs echoed across the darkened living room of the apartment. Then it happened. Darwyn felt a different kind of lust rise within him and he mournfully bowed his head as he remembered what he was.

She was beautiful and, for a short time, had made him forget about the curse that haunts him every night. But he knew that such beautiful moments could never last, they never do. This saddened Darwyn but did not stop him from what he wanted most, her life's blood.

She tilted her head back as the waves of pleasure rippled through her, completely ignorant to the monster that now lurked behind her. Darwyn caught glimpse of her throat, sweat rolling down the lovely white skin that clothed her carotid artery. He would wait no longer.

He leaned forward, sinking his cock to the hilt in her cunt, feeling her firm ass pressing against his abdomen as he pinned her to the wall. His teeth sank deep into her flesh, piercing the throbbing artery easily. She gasped, more from surprise than pain and for a moment tried to struggle but stopped as the waves or orgasm rushed through her once again. Darwyn drank deeply of her passionate blood and as he did so, began to thrust deeper into her warm depths. Once her orgasm subsided she did not resist. Instead, she gave herself completely to Darwyn, wanting more and more to feel his cum inside of her. And Darwyn would not disappoint her.

He continued to drink from her passionate, crimson well. His thrusts were becoming more urgent with each passing moment and he knew it would not be long before his lust would overtake him again. He felt her grow weak in his arms from blood loss. The time had come, he could wait no longer. With a final thrust, his cum jetted into her depths. He held her tightly as her tight cunt milked his dick of every last drop of come. He relaxed his grip and she turned to face him, a soft smile decorating her pale face. Her eyes met his and then she collapsed unconscious in his arms.

Darwyn carried her lovingly to a darkened room and an awaiting bed and layed her gently upon it. She softly opened her eyes and looked up at him in the darkness of the quiet room. For an eternity they stared at one another, caressing the soul of the other with peaceful eyes.

She knew what she had become. She had dreamed of it years before and had prayed that it would become reality ever since. It seems that dreams do come true. Her smile became broader upon her face. She knew that she would never have to leave him now and she cradled this thought affectionately and took it to sleep with her. As sleep overtook her, Darwyn strolled quietly over to the window and stared out into the sleeping city. Perhaps humans and vampires were not so different after all or perhaps it just doesn't matter.

Sèphera Girón first hooked up with the Blue Blood *crew through Cecilia Tan from Circlet Press. Circlet published an anthology called* SM Futures *which included another of Girón's stories "Shall We Dance" which takes place in the same world as "Bodie". Girón has written for all sorts of magazines all over the U.S. and Canada. Her credits include fiction and articles in* New Blood, Premiere, Videomania, Horror News, Video Industry Monthly, Videovue, Video Trade, *and* Smash. *With Julian Grant, Girón co-wrote* Creep, *a film about a creep looking for love in a night club.* Creep *won an award at the Belgium International Film Festival and Girón and her filmmaker husband (recurring motif here) have more independent features in the works.*

Bodie

by Sèphera Girón

Serena wandered along Queen street, staring into the windows of funky boutiques, wishing she had the body and the cash to parade the latest look in Goth.

Wishing wasn't going to get her the leather studded bustier or that lovely black velvet hat. More than her art work and shitty waitress job were bringing in. But the craving for money was secondary to the haunting hollow ache, a hole that never healed in her heart. The lament for love, unrequited.

Sighing, she walked along the street, her hands thrust deep into the pockets of her royal purple velvet coat. It wasn't far to the Paradise from here and she had a lifetime membership.

Adam, the multiply pierced and tattooed bouncer was at the door and she exchanged minimal pleasantries with him. He let her in through the chain link that kept out the unknowns and the voyeurs. She murmured a thanks and Adam watched her sad huddled silhouette disappear up the stairs. He was used to Serena. She always came in quiet and depressed, but a couple of hours in the Paradise usually cheered her up.

The Paradise transformed all who entered.

Serena followed the thumping of music up to the second floor, bypassing several possibilities. The Paradise was a renovated warehouse with rooms to serve a multitude in both music and the flesh. Serena made her way down a hall, passing the door to the dance cave that was open to the public.

She stopped in front of a door painted emerald green. On the lock was a computer keypad and she pressed her thumb down on it. The door buzzed open and Serena entered.

She didn't often come to this room. She told herself she found the pace too slow, that there was no loud pounding music. Her stomach flip flopped as she looked around the familiar setting. It was more like a member's lounge than a waiting room. A sparsely populated section of the club that offered rest and relaxation.

Serena hung her coat on the rack and sat down on one of the green leather couches. She closed her eyes, trying to will away the worries that plagued her. The money that trickled in was barely enough to suit her needs. She tried to nudge away the unhappiness she felt at taking a part time waitressing job to supplement her poetry, the hollow ache of having no one special to inspire her heart and mind.

Or was there?

She knew why she was here, but that was truly a dream.

She closed her eyes, wanting to let her mind open up and swallow the high sweet notes being piped into the room.

She sat like this for awhile, her mind clearing, her body relaxing. Soon she felt the lightness in her veins that came with burdens unloaded and forgotten. Her worries were safely tucked away in an unseen corner of the room.

There was a hand on her shoulder. Warm and strong, touching her firmly, but not gripping. She saw a shimmering behind her eyelids and she smiled.

"Bodie."

"Are you ready?" he asked, his voice a low resonance of rich velvet.

Serena opened her eyes and tilted her head up to look at Bodie. He was watching her with eyes as deep green as the couch where she sat. She smiled and stood up, calming the new nervousness that quivered in her bones.

"I haven't seen you here for a long time." Bodie said as he opened another green door. This one led to a small room painted a pale aqua that embraced her soul as she entered.

"I've had a lot on my mind." Serena said softly.

"But you still come to Paradise." Bodie said, smoothing a pale pink sheet across a narrow chiropractor bed.

"I keep hoping to forget." Serena said, half to herself.

"The mind body connection is very strong. You can't enjoy the yourself in the other rooms if you are cluttered." Bodie turned to her, locking his piercing jade eyes with her pale blue ones. Serena lowered her gaze guiltily.

"No matter how much you try."

His voice was stern and Serena knew that if anyone else ever scolded her that way, she wouldn't put up with it. But coming from Bodie it was more concern that she have the ultimate experience that the Paradise had to offer. It was his job. She had been avoiding the room, Bodie, it was true. But not because of the way he adjusted her bones.

She was afraid of becoming to involved in the sessions. It was his job to make the body sing, to turn away the dark clouds of despair, to soothe over aching pain with a firm hand and a quick twist.

But the last few times she had been there, she had found herself wondering what lay on the other side of his riveting eyes and warm certain hands. She found herself carrying images of his soft hair into her day time thought, and that would not do.

In a club of free sex and abandoned emotion it was not smart to become involved with the help. They did it for the money, the tips. They didn't let their emotional guard down. It would be career suicide to become emotionally attached to their clients; from bartender to dominatrix to masseuse to chiropractor. It was their job to look good and to make their clients feel better. Though Bodie had never touched her in a manner contrary to the most professional of chiropractors, the thought of his flesh touching hers in a more animal way had been haunting her for weeks. Serena clutched her hands together, all thoughts of relaxation long gone.

"I'll be right back." Bodie said, indicating the gown lying across the bed.

Serena stared at the gown for a long time. The music was a little louder now. She guessed Bodie had turned it up. He knew her so well. He knew her nervousness, the symptom, but he didn't know it's cause, the gaping hole gnawing through her.

Serena took of her clothes and stared for a moment at her soft round body. She was sadly out of shape, the way most professional writers are. At least the waitress job would keep her body active although she wasn't certain if her mind was up to the task.

She slipped on the silk gown and savored it's satin touch against her flesh.

It was wonderfully exquisite. She saw that her nipples were hard small buttons, rippling the line of the gown.

Bodie returned.

"Are you ready?" he asked. Serena nodded not meeting his eyes. If she glanced at those sparkling emeralds she would not be able to stand it. Her attempt at even the most remote stab of composure would be shattered. He was paid to touch her, to rearrange her bones. No more. No less.

Serena lay down on the bed. Bodie started to rub her back. She closed her eyes, trying not to lose herself in his warm firm touch. After this, she would definitely visit the dungeon she promised herself.

"I read your poem in *Fantasy Monthly*." Bodie said, pressing his fingers into her reluctant pelvic girdle. She winced with pain.

"What did you think?" Serena asked, remembering the tears over the tender words describing her lost love. Of a lover that had never existed for her, but of course, a poet could not admit to that. The purpose of the poem was to inspire and share the pain and loss and renewal despite what she herself might really have experienced.

"I liked it. You have a good ear for words. It reminded me of when my wife and I split up."

Serena tensed suddenly, then willed herself to relax under his hands.

"You got a divorce?" she asked. She had met Natasha once. A dark haired fire vixen that writhed on the dance floor like a burning flame. Her vibrant spirit seemed a paradox to Bodie's cool demeanor.

"A separation. A trial. Just to see."

His fingers pushed harder and Serena gasped.

"Sorry." Bodie said.

"I'm sorry. About your wife I mean."

"It's all right. Time will tell. Time always tells."

Bodie was worming his fingers up her spine now. She felt the crack and pop of each vertebrae under his touch.

"Take a deep breath in." he said. Serena sucked in.

"Now release it." Bodie said. As Serena blew out, Bodie pressed on her upper back and she felt a snap as the vertebrae clicked back into their proper places.

"Oh." Serena sighed as a wave of satisfaction calmed her.

"Feel better?" he asked.

"Much."

His fingers returned to prod her tight lower back. Sharp

pains tingled through her as he did that, trying to loosen the years of atrophy. She tried to listen to the music again, not thinking about how close his hands were to parts where they could really work some magic. Where anywhere else in Paradise they were supposed to be touching.

"You like your job here?" Serena asked.

"I like being a chiropractor. I don't know how long I'll stay at Paradise."

"You must make good money here."

"I do OK. But of course, I don't get tips like some of the other people do. I don't perform those other services."

"Have you thought about it?"

"Performing the other services?" Bodie's hands stopped for a moment. Serena started to sweat, realizing how transparent the question had been. But then the fingers started to work at her again.

"Of course I've thought about it. I'm sure Natasha thinks I've indulged in it. But, in all clear conscience, I really am a doctor. Not a sex therapist."

"Right."

"I'm thinking of getting a real office. The money wouldn't be as good at first, but..."

"Would you miss it here?"

"I would miss a lot of you. But not the weird hours. Turn over."

Serena shifted over, her gown slithering up and she pulled it back down. Her breasts flopped and she could still feel her nipples pushing towards him despite how she tried to think about other things. He was sitting at the head of the table now, massaging the back of her neck. This was the part she liked best. His hands holding her head, his fingers rubbing her neck, soothing and warm. He held her life in his hands like this. One wrong twist and she could be dead.

"I hope you don't leave. At least, for a while." Serena said softly.

Bodie adjusted her neck. First one side, and then the other. He placed her head gently on the bed.

Serena opened her eyes and looked up at him. He was staring down at her.

"You know, Serena..." he started. He licked hi lips and then stood up.

"What?" Serena sat up. Bodie had gone over to the other side of the room. If there had been a window, she was sure he would be looking out of it.

"Nothing." Bodie said. Serena felt a sadness tremble through him.

"What's wrong, Bodie?"

"I'm a good doctor, Serena. I really am. I'm younger than many that choose this profession, it's true. But I really believe in what I'm doing. However..."

"Go on..."

"Ever since I read that poem of yours. You know, it caught me off guard. I knew you wrote, but the beauty of the words...It was like you had opened up and read my heart."

"I'm sorry if I hurt you. I didn't even know about you and..."

Bodie turned suddenly and Serena saw his eyes were soft now. She had never seen them like that and her heart started to pound as she instinctively wanted to cuddle him to her breast.

I've been seeing you for well over a year, and yet I don't know you. I know many of the others so much more. You talk a lot, but not about your true self. You are guarded. Then when i read your poem, it was like a little piece of your soul had slipped out and I realized why I've been feeling so empty."

Serena stared at him. Bodie looked down at his hands.

"I'm a good doctor. Even though I work at a sex bar, I don't abuse my practice." he said again, the words sounding more like a stubborn child fessing up to an accidental broken window then a professional laying claim to his ethics.

"I'm not getting you, Bodie." Serena said. "What is so wrong?"

Bodie looked up at her and his eyes were glittering, the softness gone.

"I want you, Serena." he said. "I touch you and I try not to think about what I am doing, just finding the bone, the muscle, trying to mate them and match them and reacquaint them with each other, but it isn't working. I can't do it anymore."

"What do you want from me?"

Bodie walked back towards her and sat down on the bed beside her. He took her hand.

"I think . . . I think you want it too." he said. Serena looked at his hand wrapped around hers and nodded.

Bodie leaned towards her and pressed his lips to hers. A soft kiss, flesh barely touching. They drew back and stared at each other and this time Serena let herself drown in Bodie's eyes. He kissed her again, this time harder and she felt herself sinking back onto the table. His hands cupped her breasts, sliding on the silky gown, her nipples rocks between his fingers.

This is what I've been missing, Serena thought. The tenderness. The unexpected. God, his eyes are green.

The music washed over them, and she found herself growing lighter with every stroke of his finger. Her mind started to float, swirling with the delicious sensation of her body that seemed so far away.

She felt him touching her firmly, her arms, her legs, her back. There was a soft slithering sound as he peeled back her flesh to get at her bones. They rotated, turning under his guidance, and she felt his tongue licking along her arm bones, and over her rib cage. A soft warmth wrapped around each vertebrae in her spine, comforting and inspiring.

He tilted her stiff pelvic girdle, rotating her hips with ease, exploring the whiteness of her inner self. His tongue followed down her legs, sucking on her toes. Her sense of excitement grew as she glimpsed him through half open eyes.

Bodie lay back and Serena started to kiss his body, peeling back the layers with ease as he had done to her. She found the sensation of wrapping her tongue around his bones exquisite, and lapped at his rib cage. She worked her way down, his hands guiding her to his most urgent need.

She slid onto him, bone embracing bone. The world shimmered as she pushed against him, and she looked down at his face. He was still watching her, his forehead beading, his flesh splayed open like a picnic blanket. His breathing was hard, keeping time with hers.

She fluttered from space through time, wrapping around the music, pulsing with Bodie's energy. She was melding with his essence, a dance of tingling vibration. Their bodies met and parted on the narrow bed. She clutched at his hands, holding them above his head, marveling at the whiteness of their joints against the blue and red veins that throbbed and pulsed with their hearts. She looked at his eyes again and realized she was no longer in the chiropractor office, but somewhere else that was neither air nor water but green all around.

The sensations heightened and she was gasping his

name. He bucked against her, muscles pulsing stronger with bulging veins. Her body stiffened as did his, then with a shiver, they were wet together in a sea of green.

Serena gasped, sucking in air as if she were drowning. Slowly, her breath came in full even waves and she opened her eyes. Bodie was standing over her, watching her, his eyes dark and penetrating. She was lying on her back, her gown hiked up, her knees bent, her feet flat on the bed. She wondered if she had dreamed it all. Bodie said nothing, but she saw his face was flushed, his shirt not as neatly tucked in as it usually was.

Bodie touched her leg firmly and pushed his weight on it, causing her legs to fall to the side, cracking her lower back. It snapped loudly and she felt it give into place.

Silently, not looking at her, he put her legs back up again and did the other side. Serena closed her eyes as she groaned, still feeling the tingling seeping through her body.

"There. That should take care of you for now." he said, clearing his throat.

Serena sat up and a wave of dizziness swam through her. She saw moisture on the bed where she had been lying and realized that it had been no dream. Bodie locked eyes with her for a moment and she tried to see past the stare to his passion, but there was nothing there. He turned away.

"Thank you, Bodie." she said, watching him leave the room.

Serena dressed and paid her bill through the computer on the door. She heard Bodie turn the music down as she left.

She made her way through the palace of lies. The Paradise was always ready to serve, but it was often unexpected.

She thought of Bodie's warm firm hands and piercing eyes. Maybe, for a moment, he had enjoyed her, too.

The thought pleased her for a moment, sending a shiver down her spine as she waved good night to Adam. She made her way further down the street, trying to push Bodie from her mind.

She had tasted him. She had quite liked him, but he was not the cure for what ailed her. She wandered down Queen Street, looking for the next club to hit, the familiar hollow ache swelling up to reclaim it's hold on her once more.

I first met Sarah McKinley Oakes at a party where some hard-on with a mohawk was trying to convince me, over Oakes' protests, that he had fucked her in some anatomically implausible position. I chose to believe the lady's story and since then Oakes has been a frequent contributor of humor pieces for BLT *and the spokesmodel for* Blue Blood. *She posed for both* Blue Blood #1 *and* Blue Blood #5 *and can often be seen showing off in remarkably small outfits at the CBLT booth at science fiction conventions. A preschool teacher by day, Oakes is the ultimate woman, sensual and nurturing. Also, Oakes would like all Los Angeles-based readers to believe that everything in "Accept No Substitutes" is absolutely fictional and any resemblance to LA scenesters living or dead is purely coincidental. Mostly anyway.*

Accept No Substitutes

by Sarah McKinley Oakes

I couldn't believe the size of the place. It was huge. The biggest club back home would have fit inside of it, twice. It was two stories tall, with only a thin balcony as the second floor, where you could stand and look down on the people dancing. One entire wall was video screens, and the sound system sent music pumping through my body so hard I could barely walk. I had arranged to meet André here, but looking at the crowd I didn't know how I would ever find him. One black mohawk looks much like any other in a crowded, dark club, especially one you've never been in before.

Luckily, he was more accustomed to the place, and I soon felt his strong arms wrapping around me from behind, sending electricity shooting up and down my spine, and making my cunt ache. Damn André. We had met a week before in psych class on the first day of the semester. We got along great, laughed at all the same things, and had stayed up til three talking. We were half naked before he mentioned he had a girlfriend. I don't fuck guys with girlfriends. Even though she sounded like a real bitch, who was totally incapable of making him happy, she was still a person who didn't deserve to be cheated on. Besides, I didn't want to be a fling, I wanted him to fuck me for real. When I told him this, he said he understood and then set about doing everything he could think of to change my mind. I tried not to let on, but I was seriously weakening. No guy had turned me on as much as he did in as long as I could remember. I felt like I could come just looking at him. He was beautiful, tall with broad, strong shoulders. He had skin soft as velvet over rock hard muscles. His eyes were the color of candy kisses, he was always tan, and his brilliant smile lit up any room he was in. At night I lay in bed picturing him in my mind, and almost cried from frustration.

"You look hot. Do you want a drink?" I could barely hear him over the music, even though he was screaming in my ear, so I just nodded and let him lead me to the bar. He kept his arm around my waist as we walked and I thought about brushing it away, but couldn't bring myself to do it. We got our drinks and stood with our backs to the wall, watching the crowd. I listened to the music and pretended not to notice his hand, with was slowly sliding down my ass, and then dropping below to the backs of my thighs, rubbing the bare skin just above my stockings. A song that sounded familiar came on, and I was just trying to place it when André leaned down and yelled, "They're playing our song!" Then I heard the words 'I want to fuck you like an animal/I want to feel you from the inside.' It was "Closer to God" by Nine Inch Nails. I started moving my hips to the music and as I did André moved his hand up underneath my miniskirt. Pushing my panties out of the way, he started rubbing my pussy, brushing my clit with his thumb, occasionally almost putting his fingers inside me and then pulling back. I thought I was going to die, I wanted him so bad. I prayed nobody else could tell what was going on, and concentrated on keeping a bored expression on my face. Finally when I thought I was going to collapse, he put his mouth up to my ear and said "Do you want me to put my fingers inside you?" I knew it was wrong, and was just about to say no when I felt myself nodding. I gasped out loud when his fingers entered me, I couldn't help it, it felt so good. I don't think anyone heard, it was so loud in there and no one was paying any attention to us anyway. He moved his fingers in and out of me to the music and before I knew it I was coming. I started to fall but he grabbed me around the waist with his free hand and covered my mouth with his. It seemed like I came forever, with his fingers never slowing down for a second the whole time. Finally I knew I was done and pulled back. He took his fingers out and licked them off, then looked at me and laughed. "You are the hottest babe I know" he said with a smile, and then went off to get another drink.

I was leaning against the wall, pretty much recovered, when he returned. I figured I should be feeling guilty, but I wasn't. It had felt so good. "Let's go outside for a minute," He yelled. "I want to talk to you." Nothing makes my stomach drop quicker than a guy saying he wants to talk to me. I had a sudden urge to try and disappear into the crowd, but I figured it wouldn't work so I followed him to the door.

"I've been thinking," He said, flashing me his gorgeous smile. "I think the next best thing to fucking you myself would be hearing the details from a friend who got to fuck you. So pick out any guy in there and if I know him, I'll introduce you. What do you say?"

I stared at him, having no idea how to respond. On the one hand, I wanted him, not some friend of his. But on the other hand, I really, really needed to get laid. It had been ages. What with packing up to come to college, then getting here and finding that my place to live had fallen through, and ending up living on a friends couch for who knows how long, well, I hadn't had much chance to get fucked. I figured this might be my last chance for a while." Okay, on two conditions. One, that you only introduce me to people you know aren't insane axe murderers, and two, that you swear you aren't getting paid for this."

He laughed and pressed something into my hand, and

then turned and started walking into the club. I looked at what he'd given me. Condoms. Four of them. I followed him inside.

It took a while, but eventually I spotted the guy I wanted. Tall and lean, he was leaning against the wall talking to three other guys with an intense expression on his face. He had tilted eyes that were probably green, cheekbones you could carve wood with, and his mohawk was the same shade of purple as mine. He was as unlike André as a guy could get and still be hot. He was perfect. "That one," I told André. I started to point but caught myself just in time. "The one against the wall there. The purple one."

"Craig?" André had an amazed expression on his face. "What do you see in him?"

"Never mind that. Do you know him? Can you introduce us?"

"Of course I know him. He's Craig Night, the lead singer for Dark Nights. Hold on a second, I'll bring him over."

André was gone before I could say anything. Suddenly I was very nervous. I hoped André had the sense not to tell this guy what was up. I stared off into the crowd, not letting myself watch them, trying to appear as nonchalant as possible. It wasn't easy. Soon I felt them beside me, and looked up. "Hey Sarah, I want you to meet a friend of mine, Craig. Craig, Sarah. Sarah, Craig." As Craig and I smiled at each other, André pretended to see someone on the dance floor. "Oh, shit, I just noticed someone I have to talk to. I have to go. Call me tomorrow, okay. Good seeing you, Craig." He clapped us both on the shoulder and disappeared into the crowd. I stared after him for a second and then looked up into Craig's face, opening my eyes wide.

"I guess he forgot. He was my ride home." Craig smiled

down at me and I started to relax.

It was perfect weather for a ride in a convertible, but we decided not to put the top down because it would muss our hair. I told him where I was staying and he eased into traffic. I was thinking hard. How could I convince him to take me to his place? The couch I was using as a bed was not my idea of a good place to fuck. "So, do you live around here?" I asked, trying to sound like I was just making conversation.

"Sure, I've got an apartment about five minutes from here. It's a real nice place. Would you like to see it?" He looked at me out of the corner of his eye and smiled. That was easy.

He showed me around for about half a minute and then led me into the bedroom. It was a large room, with a huge four poster bed in the middle. He took me in my arms and kissed me, then pulled back and studied my face. "You're beautiful. I think I smudged your lipstick. What shade is that?"

"Blackberry. Revlon. Same as yours, I can tell." I traced his lips with my tongue. "You'll have to do my make-up some time. I can never get my eyeliner as perfect as yours is." He smiled at this and gently brushed my eyelid with his finger.

"All you need," He whispered as he lowered me onto the bed, "Is a very, very steady hand."

"Is there any particular brand you recommend?" I asked as I helped him undo my bra.

"The cheap ones are usually best," He answered, brushing my nipples lightly with his hand, and then moving his head down and licking them, slowly, softly. I ran my fingers through his hair and worked my hips so that my cunt was rubbing against his ribcage. He moved up to kiss me again and put his hand under my skirt, stroking my pussy through my panties, moving in slow circles. I felt the muscles in my thighs clench and drove my cunt against his hand, bucking my hips and kissing him so hard I thought my lips would bleed. As they orgasm faded, I fell back against the bed, breathing hard and looking up at the delighted expression on his face. I always feel a little embarrassed the first time I lose control in front of a guy, so to distract myself I reached down and started stroking the enormous bulge in his pants. I wanted his cock in my hands, but he was wearing so many belts around his hips there was no way I could undo them all without help. He stood up and started slowly taking them off. I wished he would hurry. I took off my bra the rest of the way and pulled my soaking panties off. I decided to leave everything else, skirt, stockings, garter belt and boots, on. Some guys like that, and I figured if he didn't he could take them off himself. When he had finally gotten all his belts off he pushed me back on the bed and fell on top of me. We kissed for a while, and then I unzipped his pants and pulled his cock free. It was huge. I wanted it inside me so bad. But not yet. I stroked it for a while, up and down, enjoying the way he moaned. Then I rolled over on top of him and kissed him, letting my satin miniskirt brush the length of it.

"I'll be right back," I told him, hopping up and finding my purse where I had left it on the floor. I eventually dug out the condoms André had given me and climbed back on the bed, only to find him already rolling one on to his dick. "Here, let me do that," I said, wrapping my lips around the head and rolling the condom down the rest of the way with my mouth. I looked up and smiled at him. He grinned and lay back, reaching down and running his fingers through my hair. He had taken off his pants while I was looking for my purse, so I was able to kiss his thighs and balls before returning to his penis. I put the head of it in my mouth and swirled my tongue around, and then pulled it out and licked up and down the underside, where that little ridge is. The muscles in his stomach started to twitch and his grip on my hair tightened. I waited until I thought he was going to come, and then rolled away.

He groaned and looked up. "Why did you stop?" I answered by climbing on top of him and rubbing my cunt against his cock. He grabbed my arms and held them behind me, then rolled over so that I was underneath him. He held my arms pinned above my head and started pushing his dick against my pussy, almost inside of me but not quite. "Do you want me to fuck you?" He asked. "Do you want it inside of you?"

"Oh god yes please," I cried, wrapping my legs around him, trying to pull him inside of me. With no warning, he shoved his cock into me, making me feel like I was going to split in two. He moved in an out, fast and hard, while I screamed and tried to rise up to him. Just as I started to come he slowed, moving his hips like a corkscrew, making my orgasm go on and on, never quite peaking, never quite ending. He pulled out long enough to turn me over onto my stomach, then went back to fucking me slowly and gently. I tried to move against him, to pick up the pace a little, but he took firm hold of my hips and held me still. When I got to the point where I knew I couldn't stand it any longer, he suddenly started going faster. Keeping one hand one my waist, he moved the other underneath me and started rubbing my clit with his fingers. The combination of his hand and his cock was unbelievable, and I started coming incredibly hard, grinding my ass into his stomach as I screamed into the bedspread. I felt him tense behind me and could tell by the way his cock jumped that he was coming too. We screamed incoherently together for awhile, and then collapsed, sweaty and exhausted.

The next day we slept late and then went out to breakfast at a diner down the block. We both said all the required stuff about how we really liked each other but didn't want a relationship, and then I hugged him good-bye and headed home.

It was only a fifteen minute bus ride from Craig's house to mine. I felt a little uncomfortable in last night's outfit. Clothes that seem perfectly reasonable when it's dark out always look ludicrous in broad daylight. It was a few blocks walk from the bus stop, and I hoped none of my neighbors were outside.

I was just approaching my house, trying to remember if I had any classes that day, and how late I'd be if I took time to change, when I saw someone on the doorstep, apparently asleep. I slowed down, not knowing what to do. It was a pretty safe section of town, but you can never be sure. I wondered if my friends were home. Maybe if I screamed they'd hear. Then I got a little closer, and saw that it was André. He sat up and looked at me for a moment, then jumped to his feet. "Sorry about that, I didn't mean to doze off, but I was up all night." He ran a hand through his mohawk, which was leaning at a crazy angle. He would have looked comical if he didn't seem so upset.

"André, what's wrong? Why are you here? Is everything okay?" I was really worried. He never goes out in public if his hair isn't perfect.

"I thought I liked the idea of knowing you were with one of my friends, but I was wrong." He was staring at the ground, talking very fast. "I nearly went out of my head I was so jealous. And I realized I want to be with you, more than anything. So this morning I went over to my girlfriends place and we broke up. I turns out she's been wanting to dump me for weeks." He looked up and smiled at me. "So what do you think? Can we give it a try?" And then I was in his arms.

I'm me and stuff and I prefer it when an editor shows her stuff, not just her taste. Some bio info on yours truly: I was born in London and raised bouncing about through Europe, the Middle East, and my fave, the US of A. My recent short fiction has appeared in the anthologies Noirotica and Power Tools, Cleis Press's Dark Angels, and the Circlet Press anthologies Blood Kiss and Sex Crime. Collaborating with Blue Blood art director Forrest Black, I co-wrote a great deal of Destiny's Price, White Wolf's street-culture sourcebook. Over one hundred humor pieces of mine have seen print in markets ranging from Chic to Key DC to my own humor zine BLT. During the late eighties, I wrote about a billion rock journalism pieces for publications including Hit Parader, Rock Scene, and Concert Shots (plus a bunch of dishonest local newspapers who never paid their bills). And, as you have probably all figured out by now, I edit Blue Blood. Recently, I have been making a thorough study of sushi bars in Georgia and taking lots of photographs of naked people. Although I don't think these two passions are causationally related, you never know. Y'all can reach me down south these days c/o Blue Blood.

Dreamgirl

by Amelia G

You probably know him from his solo career, rather than what came first. Before the platinum years, Wesley Acton was in a more theatrical band called False Witness. They had all the cheesy nineties stuff — devil worship, Charles Manson samples, on-stage whippings and all sorts of weird fetishistic ritualism . . . or maybe it was ritualistic fetishism. Whichever. At any rate, they had the necessary stage presence and they were good too. I mean, really good.

The night that it either all came together or all fell apart (depending upon your perspective), Wes was in no mood for a woman. They'd just done two nights in Chapel Hill and he'd convinced himself that he kind of liked the girl he'd hooked up with there — delicate little Goth creature, not his usual type. Maybe he actually did like her or maybe he'd just been on tour for too many weeks in a row. Or maybe it had something to do with certain abilities to remove chrome from a trailer hitch, as they say in the small town in rural Georgia where Wes grew up. So Wes told the little suction cup that he'd like to call her when False Witness came back through town supporting Slayer on the Dark Servants tour.

"Slayer?" she sniffed. "Aren't they metal or something? I think I fucked their drummer once."

"You think? You don't know?"

"Oh, honey." She smiled pityingly as she slid her palm down his chest towards his crotch again. "Girls don't fuck boys in touring bands 'cause they want a relationship so bad."

So Wes Acton was in no mood for a woman when he and the rest of False Witness arrived in Atlanta. It was November and unseasonably cold for Georgia, but there were already girls hanging out outside The Wreck Room when the band members began carrying the equipment in from the van. The groupies variously wore leather and PVC and a smattering of latex. The girls either had sleek glossy hair in some moderately natural color or else they had horribly damaged but fantastically colorful plumage flying wildly about their shoulders. Some sported pentagram necklaces and cut-off concert T-shirts, and the other bands they liked (and were admitting to at the time) were Electric Hellfire Club and Deicide. "I want to kiss your cruel mouth!" one minimally leather-clad vixen screamed.

"She talking to you or me?" Caine asked Wes.

"I don't think I have a 'cruel mouth', so it must be you."

"Wish she'd help me carry the damn keyboards."

Neither Wes nor Caine could really believe that there could be significant numbers of girls who were actually attracted to them. Caine had been a scrawny junior high boy. With bad acne. Now, the keyboardist was a few years older and he was the member the groupies called "the good-looking one." (Although you were a more important starfucker even then, if you had Wes in your portfolio.) Caine's pasty skin was acne-scarred, but there were no current conflagrations. He was still painfully skinny, but the pitch-black hair half-way down his back was enough to win their hearts. Or at least their mouths.

Wes was of the opinion that he and Caine looked like Abbott and Costello after they met the Mummy, Frankenstein, and Satan. Really, Wes was stocky but not fat. With his short curly dark brown hair and homemade stage costumes, the girls compared Wes to Mel Gibson in "The Road Warrior" much more often than to any long-dead comedic fat boys. He was always dressed for the apocalypse and he had these absolutely chilling huge blue eyes and a football player's body. He had actually played football in ninth grade before the incident with Mindy.

If Wes had not met Mindy, he knew he might have mainstreamed. His whole life might have been different. Maybe it wouldn't have mattered how his father had been. Maybe his mother would have lived. Maybe he would have been there to save her. But that is not the way it went. He did meet Mindy.

Mindy had been the town doctor's overweight bookish daughter. She tried to dress like the other girls in their class, but her drab brown hair had been permed too tightly and the pastel clothing accentuated her weight problem and the whole look just did not work on her. In his teens, Wes' adult look was already beginning to push its way through to the surface of the chubby boy with chipmunk cheeks and glasses. Mindy had been quietly attracted to Wes from the time she passed puberty, but now with his improved looks and her own raging blossoming hormones, she craved him. She was prepared to do anything to get him.

Wes had made a childhood show of dabbling with the occult, a creepy kid really, he always had his nose in a book by Aleister Crowley or Anton LaVey or else he was reading yet another true account of some serial killer's rampage. After he was found with Mindy came the gray institution years. They wouldn't let him have any of his precious books in here. They said the books were part of how come he was sick.

They asked about his parents, and they said it was very important that he be honest. Wes told them how his father used to hit him with his belt for being such "a fat disgusting slob" and the doctors told Wes that he would get out sooner if he didn't lie so much. Wes told them how his father had slapped his mother around saying she must have fucked some fat guy, because Wes sure couldn't be his kid. And the doctors would sigh because they feared they were wasting their time with someone who would never have a good mind again. When Wes protested that it was the truth, they prescribed sedation and shook their heads for they feared Wes would never never get well. So he spent nearly three gray years inside the institution walls, years warmed only by his dreams of a girl of flame. At the time, it would have seemed incredible to Wes that someday there would be more girls in his life, more than just a dream girl. But then, as Caine liked to say girls were the second, third, and fifth best reasons to get into rock and roll. (The first best was loving the music and the fourth was the free drugs.)

So, that night in Atlanta, Caine was ogling the girls who had come out to see False Witness. He kept telling them that his name was "Caine, Mr. Hugh Mongus Hardcock if you're nasty." Caine had roadied for Janet Jackson for a while and he thought this line was about the funniest thing anyone had ever thought of saying, much less had the nerve to say.

Wes was feeling crabby, but he had to admit that the groupies in Atlanta were always the hottest. Growing up in the boonies, he'd heard that Atlanta had seventy-five strip clubs in the city proper and he believed it. Caine kept pointing out this girl or the other and they were all undeniably appealing, but then Caine spotted one sweet thing who was so incredible Wes thought perhaps he was in the mood for a woman after all. Her hair was the exact same shade of red as the Coke cans at the Coca-Cola Museum in downtown Atlanta, which False Witness had made the pilgrimage to that afternoon. (Caine liked to joke about how the journey to the Coca-Cola Museum was the only thing the band was religious about, but his brother contended that Satanism was too a religion. And Wes just tried not to consider the question at all.) The girl had a shock of lemon yellow hair streaking up the side of her head on either side, bride of Frankenstein style. She wore red fishnets on her long legs and over them a shiny red PVC mini- skirt which hung low on her hips showing off her muscular abdomen. Above the waist, she wore only a gold slave chain which hung loosely below her navel and what looked like red gaffer's tape hiding the nipples on her shockingly buoyant breasts. With all the strip clubs in Atlanta, tit jobs were tremendously common, but Wes didn't care if a stripper's tits felt like bags of gravel to the touch because most of them were awfully nice to look at. He imagined that this red-haired girl's breasts would feel as good as they looked and he wanted to bury his cock between those gorgeous gifts to mankind, no matter what.

Wes and Caine's attention was called away from the ogling department when the promoter came up to introduce himself. Well, really he came up to tell them they were going on stage later than had been expected. The guy said his name was Jeff Ray and there was some band going on before False Witness on account of how that band had been willing to pay to play.

After Jeff Ray wandered off, Caine commented that they ought to make up some nice rhyming lyrics with Ray and pay and play.

"There was something wrong with that guy," said Wes, "like his head was too little for his body or something."

"If you say so." Caine shrugged. Now that he thought about it, he guessed Jeff Ray did have a weirdly weasely little face for such a big jock sporto guy body. Caine, however, was much more interested in checking out the female half of the population and the doors had just opened so he figured they only had a few hours until showtime. And Caine wanted to line up company before the show.

Wes meanwhile went off to try to convince the bartender to give him a drink. At age twenty, he was closer to being of age than Caine or their guitarist Ralph or their temporary drummer, this weightlifter chick Dragon. But closer wasn't good enough to get him a drink at the Wreck Room. He wanted the drink or six on account of how any show in Georgia always made him nervous. The town he grew up in was awfully far out in the middle of fucking nowhere, but an Atlanta show still felt like a hometown show and there was always the chance that Mindy would show up. Not that it was likely, given that Wes had heard she married some accountant and settled down to push out babies in the town where she and Wes grew up. She hadn't had to deal with the stigma he had. People had, if anything, been nicer to her afterwards because she had been perceived as a victim.

Although Wes had been judged totally responsible for the Mindy debacle, the whole thing had been her idea really. He supposed that he knew the girl had a crush on him, but it hadn't really occurred to him at the time that doing a ritual was her idea of flirting, her hope of making time with him. Wes had not processed that she was trying to summon a sex demon for a reason. Wes had, however, found her almost attractive in the big black robe she sewed herself for the occasion. He had been touched that she had made him one too. And it had been Mindy who used the scalpel stolen from her dad's home office. They had done the ritual at Wes' home while his father was out and his mom was zonked out on sleeping pills. Perhaps the authorities had felt Wes was the instigator partly because they did not do it at Mindy's place.

At any rate, the idea had been to do a summoning and the really creepy part was that both Mindy and Wes had thought it worked at the time. Later Wes had come to see that the psychiatrists were right, but in a weird way, he had always wondered if maybe the magic would have worked right (instead of fucking up his life) if Mindy had not cut so deep. Then again, it was right before he passed out that he had come and the room had seemed to shimmer with something mystical.

Mindy had insisted that it was an important part of the ritual for Wes to let her touch his penis. She said that a succubus had to be bound to an earthly location by a man's sperm. That way the man could control her even if they crossed the barriers of any protective circle. And what is the point of summoning a sex demon, if you can't break the circle to touch it. "That way," Mindy said, "the demon gets trapped on our plane and in our general geographical area and she can't leave until you say." And Mindy had given Wes a look that was less seductive than she intended, but still terribly promising from Wes' perspective.

They had lit dozens of black candles and sticks of incense in Wes' room. The smoke was so thick in the small bedroom that it was difficult to see. Wes thought Mindy looked better slightly out of focus, smoother, softer in a good way. And she had drawn various symbols on the floor in chalk and generally acted like she knew what she was doing, although Wes did not recognize most of it from any of his occult books. And then Mindy had cut herself in similar patterns, drawing her black robe up and taking the scalpel to first one pudgy thigh and then the other. And that was when she reached under Wes' robe and fed his already hard cock through the flap in his white BVD's. She crawled under his robe with her big head of frizzy permed hair and kind of licked his thigh. She wanted to do more. She wanted to lick his . . . she wanted to lick Wes' thing. But she had an idea that there was a way you were supposed to do that and she didn't really know what it was, so she just licked one fuzzy thigh.

Then she had wanted to use the scalpel on Wes too. And he had let her. After all, she was touching his dick and he had never gotten a girl to do that before. She traced little red patterns along his arms and legs and across his soft tummy. It hadn't really hurt because the scalpel was so sharp and she kept touching him between his legs and everything smelled like jasmine incense and sulfurous smoke from the tallow candles and he was scared he was going to come too fast and spoil her ritual.

But then Mindy took off her robe and drew deeper and deeper curving interlocked bloody patterns across the front of her naked body. And then she dropped the scalpel and danced around the room, rubbing the blood all over her body with both hands, squeezing her small conical breasts and rubbing her voluptuous hips and ass. Wes was dumbfounded, excited, terrified his mother was going to wake up or his father was going to get home. He could even see Mindy's private parts. And he wanted to touch himself to finish it while he watched this wild dance, but he was too shy.

And Mindy used her own blood to fingerpaint crimson designs all over his floor and then she put her hand between his legs again. She didn't do it exactly the way Wes liked, not quite the way he would have done it himself. But it was more than sufficient and he came shaking, his come pooling in the middle of a large, unevenly scrawled, bright red circle Mindy had drawn on the floor. And just before he lost consciousness, the room had seemed to shimmer, to fade in and out of existence. And he thought he almost saw the form of a beautiful woman take shape in the air over that protective circle. But when he tried to focus his eyes on her, to take in her exact appearance, he found that he could not make her shape fully resolve. At the time, he thought he couldn't focus his eyes and finally passed out from coming so hard, but the doctors later told him it was from a combination of blood loss and smoke inhalation. Apparently, he'd lost a lot of blood, although not as much as Mindy who was in critical condition for three days.

Really it had been a fabulous intense experience and Wes would have looked forward to seeing Mindy again when he got out of the institution. If he hadn't lost three years of his life because of her, that is. Mindy's father had been insane with rage and hurt and he had insisted that the whole sick thing must have been Wes' idea. Wes had trouble disagreeing for a few reasons. First of all, Mindy had told the authorities that everything had been Wes' idea from the very start and she had strongly implied that he had forced her. Second, Mindy's family members were pillars of the community and his just were not. Third, as soon as he got home from the hospital which stitched him up, his father took one look at the hospital bill and beat Wes senseless. And, fourthly, Wes had been so excited by the whole interaction with Mindy; he was embarrassed; he just did not have what it took to get up in front of a room full of people and say that actually a girl all convinced him to do something like that. Besides, Wes figured that being committed meant that he would get away from his father. Which was true in a way, but three years is a terribly long time when you are a teenager, and the doctors seemed to have no idea what to do with Wes. So when he dreamed, he had not dreamed of Mindy; he had dreamed of a fantasy girl who kept him warm and whispered that she understood what he truly desired. And some nights the dream girl would do some of the things she knew he wanted, acts which he had only quite recently begun to even imagine. And the following morning the orderlies would tease Wes because they didn't really care if he ever got well.

They let Wes out after his father killed his mother. Wes figured it was primarily out of embarrassment given that they had always assumed he made up the stuff about his father's violent temper. Still, Wes figured it was no great shakes spending a year bouncing from one foster family to the next, especially when he had to go in to the institution every other week in order to be evaluated. The constant reminder of those three gray years did nothing to assist him in getting past them.

But after a year of flipping burgers at Johnny Rockets and hanging out at local clubs, Wes had gotten away from the rotation of foster parents and psychological profiles and he met Caine in a group house they both lived in and Wes didn't really know how to sing, but he had incredible stage presence and he was willing to make a spectacle of himself. And Caine and Caine's brother Ralph seemed to have a clue about making music. So False Witness was born and they moved to New York, but they tried to tour as often as possible. So they ended up in Atlanta from time to time and the whole state of Georgia made Wes feel squidgy, but he couldn't get the bartender at The Wreck Room to give him a drink.

Caine, on the other hand, had way better luck with the bartender (he found a date who was of age) and was thoroughly plowed by the time they were set to go on. At which point in time, Jeff Ray the promoter came over and told them it was going to be another hour and a half before False Witness could play because the pay-to-play warm-up had been doing sound check while Wes had been trying to get drunk and Caine had been succeeding. Not that the warm-up's set sounded much better than their supposed sound check.

Caine introduced two brunette girls with huge breasts whose names were Shawna and Kelly. "They're dancers," he said, "they're over twenty-one."

At first Wes thought that Caine had brought the two girls over so Wes could have one, but then he realized that Caine felt there was entirely enough of his skinny self to go around. Looking out for Wes' best interests, however, Caine did inquire as to whether Wes had seen anything he liked. "There was that girl with the Coke can red hair with the yellow stripes on the side . . ."

"The one with no shirt on? Just like red tape or something on her tits?"

"Yeah."

"Wes, you are a freak," Caine told him as he caressed Shawna's ass through her black mini-dress (or maybe it was Kelly's ass.) "That girl, Wes, she looks okay from the front, but she's got like these scars on her back. They're sick-looking; she's got this — this tattoo covering most of her back, big, big back piece to hide them — the scars that is — or something, but they still look fucked-up. Fucking horrible."

But when False Witness finally did get to go on-stage and do their set, the red-haired girl was in the front, right beneath the low stage, like she knew which was the only part of the floor the singer could really see to past the powerful stage lights. Wes was singing for all he was worth, despite the horribly adjusted sound board, despite the concrete block acoustics of The Wreck Room. He wanted to perform for this incredible girl who was writhing sensuously as she danced around the floor beneath him. Wes sang False Witness' ode to serial killers and he watched the girl's hips move, sliding back and forth under her shiny red miniskirt. The gold slave chain winked metallically in the changing lights as it shimmied around and around on her taut waist.

And her breasts. They were heartbreaking, impossible breasts, the sort Wes wanted to bury his face in and hide from the world. The sort Wes wanted to bury his cock in until he spurted hot come on her pouting and no-doubt receptive lips. Performing for a decent-sized crowd (which False Witness always attracted for Atlanta shows) always got Wes hot. Normally the band actually had an even bigger crowd than The Wreck Room could hold, but The Masquerade, where they would normally play, had been booked by a big national act already for the only night they could really afford to be in town, what with their other tour dates and all. But the girl in red's breasts more than made up for the smaller crowd. Wes couldn't believe that anything that size could defy gravity like that, but they were not lumpy; this girl's breasts were big and flawlessly rounded, high and proud on her chest. And Wes could see a little bit of black work on her shoulders, some tribalistic design which was no doubt part of the tattoo Caine had mentioned, but he couldn't see any horrible scars or anything like that. Not that it is easy to pick up details by club light. When they did the S&M number where Caine wears the horns and whips members of the audience, the girl raised her hand to volunteer, but Wes chose other girls over her; he wanted her for himself and, rather than looking disappointed, she smiled at him knowingly. He wondered if she could tell he was half hard in his pants just looking at her.

Wes was not left wondering for very long after the show. Ralph was arguing with the promoter about the money they were owed and the promoter was screaming about how they didn't deserve even the amount he was paying because False Witness served evil. "Oh, like you didn't know, like the band name wasn't a tip-off," Ralph was screaming back. Caine, on the other hand, was making out with Shawna and Kelly. At least Wes was pretty sure they were the same two girls. Dragon, their temporary fill-in drummer, was hanging out with a couple of obvious dykes. Wes still had her figured for straight, but Caine who had tried and failed to get into her pants was convinced the skin basher was definitely a lesbian and refused to listen when Wes said, "I think they're just her friends. And fans maybe."

At any rate, the promoter was handing Ralph about eight hundred dollars less than what the band calculated they were owed and Wes was about to go over to the bar and help Ralph scream at the weasely rip-off artist, when the girl approached him. She didn't say hello or say anything else by way of introduction; she just reached out and took one of Wes' hands and placed it on her right breast like she knew that was what he craved. Her breast felt exactly the way he imagined it would, resilient and smooth. Wes was instantly the rest of the way hard and he irritated himself by blushing, but he was a big boy, so he dropped his hand down past the sweat-sticky PVC and pressed his fingers up beneath her miniskirt. She wore no underwear and her cunt was completely hairless. She was already wet and ready for him, and his index finger slid in effortlessly. Wes looked around for a moment, but they were off to one side behind the stage and he didn't think anyone could see them, not clearly anyway. Irrelevantly, he suddenly remembered that scene in that "History of the World" movie where the French guy walks around the royal gardens sticking his hands beneath women's skirts and saying, "Ah, it's good to be the king!"

The girl was sweaty from dancing and the smell of her was musky and feminine. She pressed her hips against his finger and he slipped a second digit into her impossibly hot sex. She moaned huskily and when he dragged the ball of his thumb from side to side over the spot where he approximated her clit to be, she made a little mewling animal noise and closed her eyes. He pressed his fingers in and out of her a couple of times marveling at her wetness and how smooth her hairless mound felt. When he ran his thumb briskly back and forth again, he felt her vaginal walls spasm against his hand like her body was trying to suck him in and the expression on her face was so sexy, Wes thought that there was nothing in the world he wanted to do more than get this girl some place where he could fuck her properly.

"Let's go outside," she breathed, her whisper hot in his ear.

"I should probably help Ralph with the promoter first," Wes told her, glancing guiltily toward where the heated discussion was taking place by the bar. "That Jeff Ray fuck is ripping us off."

"Take care of it later," she murmured, and she took Wes by the hand and led him out the backstage door.

The late night November air gave him goosebumps and Wes said, "maybe this isn't the best place; you could come back to the motel with us."

"I want you now," she snarled, "now!" And then she purred, "I'll keep you warm."

"If you're not cold with no shirt on . . ."

And her kiss was hungry and demanding and Wes rubbed his crotch against her and forgot entirely about the cold. When he put his arms around her, her back felt uneven to the touch. Where the rest of her skin was springy, her back had deep jagged grooves in it on each shoulder blade.

"What happened to you?" he asked softly.

"You chained me," she answered, her breath once again hot in his ear," maybe if I'm very good, if I'm everything you ever dreamed, maybe you can set me free."

And maybe Wes would have asked questions, but she slid down his body and pulled the zipper on his black jeans down with her teeth and he didn't want her mouth occupied with anything but his grateful cock. She undid the button with her hands and slid his pants and his black washing machine-dyed BVD's down to his ankles. When she put it in her mouth, Wes asked if she wanted to use a condom for safety's sake, but he couldn't make out her reply with his dick in her mouth and she didn't take it out.

She leaned him against the brick wall in the alley and she sucked him deep into the heat of her mouth. Her mouth was wet and hot so hot and it felt like he must be thrusting halfway down her throat, but she just bobbed her head enthusiastically. And then she rubbed his member, still damp from her mouth, in between her incredible breasts. She just kept getting hotter until he imagined he could see the steam rising off of her body. Wes tangled his hands in her red hair and watched the back of her head rising and falling over his groin. Glorying in the intense sensations flooding him, he looked down her body from her strong, if admittedly pretty messed-up looking shoulder blades, caressed her back with his eyes and then admired the way her ass looked firm beneath the red PVC miniskirt which was stretched tight in her crouching position. She was licking the head of his cock and rubbing her breasts on the sides and he thought that even the scars on her back looked okay set off by that tribal style black work back piece. He wondered if she had had the tattoo done locally. The designs reminded him of something he couldn't quite pin down. And he couldn't wait to see what she looked like drenched in his come.

Abruptly she grabbed the base of his cock tightly, twisting just the tiniest bit, effectively cutting off his incipient orgasm. Wes couldn't think of anything to say but "ow."

"I want you to fuck me, fuck me," she whispered hoarsely, running her palms up under his T-shirt and dragging her long red-lacquered nails lightly across his broad rib cage on the way back down. Her nails tickled slightly and he giggled.

"I mean it," she said and Wes almost lost it with terror when she pulled out the knife. First because he couldn't figure out where she could have hidden a dagger that size and second because of what he feared she would do with it. She shook her head impatiently and put a hand between her own thighs. She pulled up the skirt so that Wes could watch her rub her naked pussy. "The knife is for me," she explained. "I need you to believe that I'm what you hope for. I need you to reopen my scars. I need you put your cock in me. I need you, you, you so bad." She was moaning now as she worked herself.

She handed Wes the knife and turned around on the ground and got down on all fours. "I'm not really comfortable with violence," Wes groaned uncomfortably. He knew this was a scene Caine would have had no problem with, but Wes' father had left him with a distaste for personal violence and there was a reason it was Caine who used the whip during their S&M songs.

"That's good, that's good," she told him as she wriggled her hips expectantly. "I need you to believe you are setting me free not hurting me. I need you to open the wounds but not cut too deep. I want your trust. Not your aggression."

"My love?" Wes distrusted groupies who said anything too strong too fast. It was like they assumed they knew him just because they knew his music. When her only reply was to spread her legs wider and tilt her ass higher in the air, Wes asked again, "My love?"

"I already have that," she laughed, a beautiful, high, tinkling laugh, "I've had it for years. And you'll have the entirety of mine when the music is truly yours."

And then his dick got the better of him and the next thing he knew he was sliding into her and she was so hot. It was a moment before he realized what her repeated instructions to, "do it now, do it now" meant. He pressed all the way into her with his cock. Then carefully, carefully he drew the dagger along the line of first one marked shoulder blade and then the other. He pressed deep enough to draw blood, but not deep enough to damage muscle or anything. If he hadn't wanted her so badly . . . but well he did want her so badly.

She came almost immediately after he cut her. He tossed the knife aside as soon as his task with it was complete, heard it clatter on the asphalt, and rubbed his palms down her body from her shoulders to her hips, the blood from his incisions smearing across her dark inscrutable tattoo, obscuring it. She bucked against his hips and her cunt was squeezing him in a perfect fit. He held onto her hips and she reared back against him, slamming backwards to meet each thrust.

She was so hot and so wet and she seemed so excited that it was Wes fucking her. Just when he knew he couldn't hold back any longer, she cried out, "don't come yet, don't come yet, don't come yet."

"What?" Wes' voice came out a yelp.

"Make me come again and you can come on my face," she moaned in between thrusts, "I know you want it that way."

And somehow he found the strength to hold off while she trembled in his grasp and her sex spasmed over his. He didn't think of football or anything like that; he just thought of how much he wanted to please this girl who knew just how to please him. And when she was done, she crawled forward and as he slipped out, she rolled over under him and drew him forward over her by pulling on his twitching cock. She laid his member down between her beautiful breasts with the nipples still encased in gaffer's tape, and she guided his hands over to touch her breasts and she squeezed them together on either side of his penis. She lifted her head up off the ground and flicked her tongue forward to lick the head again, but the position proved awkward so she rubbed the glans with the forefingers of both hands as her palms pressed her breasts against his cock and Wes looked at her full smiling lips, with the sexy pouting lower lip, and her eyes were sparkling expectantly and when his burning white come jetted across her face, she seemed to revel in it.

Maybe it was the intensity of his orgasm that made him overlook them, or maybe it was just that at that late hour in the alley behind The Wreck Room they were the same color as the dark asphalt. Whatever it was, Wes didn't notice the big black leathery wings sprouting from her back as she lay there, until one of the girls with Caine screamed from where the three of them had been watching from the backstage door.

And then Caine was bitching Wes out for not helping

settle the money problem with the promoter.

"Yeah, and how long were you watching me and, uhm . . . how long were you watching in your efforts to assist with our little promoter problem?" Wes was struggling with his pants and trying to seem in control of this argument at the same time. In his favor, he almost pulled it off.

"Fuck you," said Caine, his silhouette trembling in the doorway, "that Jeff Ray guy is fucking big."

Wes could see the two girls standing by Caine in the dim light. From what he could see of their faces, they looked bored. Wes wondered which one had just screamed, but neither showed much emotion of any kind. When he looked around for his dream girl, she was no where to be seen. From the disinterested looks on Caine's bimbo pick-ups, Wes could almost believe he had dreamed it all.

"No, Caine," he said, "fuck you!" And in his head Wes was kicking himself for not having a wittier rejoinder than that. But he was still dizzy from his orgasm and it totally pissed him off that Caine might be watching him. It was typical of Caine to act like False Witness was his own personal band when it was time to write music or anything like that, but when it came time to do the annoying tasks, then everyone was supposed to be a team.

Wes and Caine might have come to blows, or more likely might have yelled "fuck you" at one another a bunch more times, if Ralph hadn't come out the door behind Caine and Shawna and Kelly just then. "Dragon is staying with a friend tonight and I am going to the room at the Motel 6. Anyone who wants to come with me is welcome. As far as the receipts for tonight go, we are fucked and I've had enough." Wes and Caine might have continued bickering then anyway, except that Ralph commented to Caine, "Hey, that's really thoughtful; you brought enough for the whole class."

So, forgetting to be pissed at Wes, Caine started telling his brother that maybe if he dressed a little cooler and had a little respect, women would like him better. And then Shawna and Kelly decided that they had had enough fucked up weirdness, so they left and then Caine was really mad at Ralph.

The two brothers were still at each other's throats when the band members arrived at the Motel 6. They had two rooms with two single beds in each, but Wes had a room to himself because Dragon was supposed to be taking up the other one. They went into the brothers' room first and Wes walked through the adjoining door and wandered through his darkened motel room. When he went to the bathroom and turned the light on, he noticed what looked and — ouch! — felt like burn blisters on the shaft of his dick. He was standing there horrified as he examined himself when he heard her voice calling to him from the darkened bedroom. "If you love something, set it free; when it comes back to you, it's yours." She had a sweet southern twang to her voice when she spoke above a whisper.

"Let me kiss it and make it better," she crooned, "I just didn't want anyone else to touch it." And she was right, her mouth was like a cool sweet salve as he looked down at her now unscarred and untattooed back and he thought that perhaps he had seen the pattern of that disappeared tatt on a bedroom floor once a long time ago.

"You make me whole," she whispered as she lay snuggled next to him afterwards, and in the morning he was whole too. Ralph was still asleep when Caine found Wes encircled in her dark wings. And Caine was not mollified by the envelope with the eight hundred dollars in it.

"Playacting that servant of a Dark Lord shit to get girls is one thing," he sputtered, "but this is something else altogether."

Probably Ralph never believed his brother when Caine talked about it later. At first Wes found it difficult to create music without Caine and without the unnamed yearning he had suffered with for six years. But then he found a different place to sing from and that's where those wildly popular fierce love songs, the ones you would have heard of came from.

And Caine would rant to any interviewer who would listen about how this girlfriend of Wes' got eight hundred bucks they were owed out of this promoter. When the interview would ask what was so bad about that, he would exclaim, "she said she gobbled him up, she gobbled him up. And then he took his girl to meet his father. Wes took his girlfriend to meet his father." And the interviewers would sigh because they feared they were wasting their time with someone who would never have a good band again.

After the first Wes Acton album went triple platinum, of course Wes gave a lot of interviews, but when asked about why False Witness broke up, he merely cited creative differences. And odds are good, you've only seen the interviews with the guy whose solo career flourished. So that's really all there is to it.

When I first met Andrew Greenberg, he was the vampire developer for White Wolf. This meant that he was literally in charge of developing the line of vampire supplements and source material for Vampire: The Masquerade. *But, taken out of context, "vampire developer" sure does make for the coolest business card ever, plus it means that Greenberg has writing and/or development credits on more than fifty White Wolf books. He also helped design White Wolf's* Rage *card game and the* Jyhad *card game which White Wolf created in partnership with Wizards of the Coast the publishers of Magic: The Gathering. (Note:* Jyhad *is now called* Vampire: The Eternal Struggle, *after* White Wolf Corporate Politics: The Eternal Struggle -- *I mean, so that players of White Wolf's Vampire roleplaying game could better identify the card game as associated.) Within twenty-four hours of our acquaintance, Greenberg took me to Guys and Dolls, a coed strip club in the heart of Atlanta, Georgia, where we alternated between the male and female dance stages. A totally hot female stripper named Onyx set my stockings on fire while doing a table dance involving flash paper for us. Following the success of the* Dracula Unleashed *CD-ROM game which Greenberg co-wrote with White Wolf's werewolf developer Bill Bridges, Greenberg became a partner in the successful CD-ROM publishing empire that is HDI. This talented boy has even written for the* BLT *humor zine. Just make sure he never follows you into the bathroom at a club.*

Not Another Groupie

by Andrew Greenberg

As Taut Ones came to the end of its first set, Jessie began scanning the crowd, looking for a likely candidate for tonight's fun and games. The light man dimmed the stage lights on the last song, and even as he sang Jessie enjoyed the anticipation as his eyes adjusted to the dark.

He had already scoped out the legion of young man-boys crowded around the front of the stage, and at least one or two of them might do, but so far he had seen nothing special. From his vantage point at the front of the stage he could see a bevy of young ladies crowded around stage right, and Jessie dismissed them without as much as a glance. The usual cluster of daters and heteros stood in the center of the club, and Jessie saw nothing of interest among them.

Then, as he flicked one long strand of black curly hair away from his eyes, he saw just the thing, hidden against the wall to stage left. Indeed, Jessie had almost glanced right past him, and only the way the house lights had reflected off a steel gauntlet had caught his attention. As his song came to its morbid close, Jessie fixed his gaze on this tasty morsel.

The object of his attentions was tall, his lanky frame topped by closely shorn blond hair. Even from the stage Jessie could tell that he was wearing makeup which lightened his complexion, but his face still had a dark cast to it. All his clothes were black, and metal shone all over him. He couldn't be older than 23 and probably wasn't even that. The only things Jessie couldn't see were his eyes, but those never mattered.

Between sets Jessie sat in the break room, wiping his face lightly with a white hotel towel and sipping from a whiskey and coke. Club workers came and went, sometimes talking to the rest of the band but always avoiding him. No matter how much they might want to be near him, no matter how deep their desire for his hard white body, none would approach him. Only his band stayed near him, and even it rarely talked to him.

The other members of Taut Ones objected when he changed the song list for the next set, but one sneer silenced them. Jessie wanted something more driving than his usual run of slow depression, something that would get his young target pumped and energized. He knew there was little chance the blond would leave between sets. He had the look of someone who would die before leaving a show early, preferring to stay and judge both it and its audience over all else. Aloof and controlled, blondie was in it for the long haul.

As Taut Ones went on for the second set, Jessie smiled when he saw that his target was still in the exact same place. As the set continued, he began directing his songs toward that side of the club. He would stand, one strong leg propped on his monitor, and wrap his microphone cord around his muscled biceps. For the second set he had changed from his ruffled black blouse into an old cut-up band shirt, and he had unbuttoned the top of his old Levis, letting it rest on his hips. He frequently ran his left hand under the bottom of his shirt, pushing it up as he rubbed his washboard-like stomach.

For its encore, Taut Ones did Jessie's favorite pick-up song, "Nightshade." He had already instructed Karl, the band's roadie, to drop one of the band's special backstage passes next to the blond, and he directed "Nightshade," with all its cries for romance and death, right where the young man had been standing. As the song came to its morbid conclusion and the house lights came up, a thin smile crossed Jessie's lips when he saw the blonde boy standing there, fingering the ultrawhite pass. Jessie went backstage, quickly wiped the sweat from his pale body and then sat down, somewhat apart from the other members of the band.

The club had a loose policy about letting people backstage, and a steady steam of fans came through. Jessie ignored them as they stood across the room from him, but the weight of their stares relaxed him. He could feel their eyes and whispers, and reveled in the power he knew he held over them. No one else could grab an audience this jaded and force it to worship him. Let the magazines spread their sycophantic praise of bands like Last Despair and singers like Louis Debris. Others might pretend to have the attitude, but Jessie knew that only his was not an act.

Jessie himself had eyes for no one but tonight's target. He thought he caught a couple of glimpses of his blond attractor, but as the fans and members of the band paired (and sometimes tripled) up, he began to worry. Then Jessie saw him, standing alone next to the bathroom.

Jessie smiled, rose slowly from his seat and walked over to the small bathroom. Pointedly ignoring his target, he pushed the door open, looked in and then turned to the blond. "It's all right. There's nobody in there. You're free to piss as much as you like," he sneered.

Jessie half expected to startle the blond with this, and was slightly disappointed when the boy just nodded and walked into the bathroom. As the door closed, Jessie felt a cold anger grow in him, and as soon as he heard a spray of urine hit the toilet water, he opened the door. He felt his anger rise when the blond did nothing more than turn his head to see who had come in.

Unsure of what to do next and having planned to take advantage of the expected shock when he came in, Jessie stood still for a second. Then he moved up right behind his target.

"You're not doing it right," Jessie said as he moved his right hand in front of the blond. "Can't you even piss correctly?" he asked, and his right hand found the blond's hands. He slowly grasped the cock.

The blond did nothing to resist Jessie and went on urinating. Jessie began stroking the cock as he drew himself up against his target. Jessie's own dick was beginning to stir, but nothing seemed to affect the blond. Then, suddenly, the boy said, "I'm done. Shake it."

Jessie froze, then let go of the blond as if the boy were on fire. He backed up, his eyes blazing hate, before he got control of himself. The blond turned and zipped his black leather pants. Jessie saw no change in the blond's expression, but for the first time he saw the cold, pale blue eyes. They seemed to drain the anger right out of him. As the blond headed for the door, however, the anger came back redoubled.

Jessie shut the door with one hand and pointed to the sink with the other. "Wash," he commanded, feeling slightly better for having caught the blond in this omission and then feeling worse for having needed this to restore his confidence.

The blond stopped, turned back to the faucet and ran some water over his hands. Jessie again came up directly behind him and stared at the face reflected in the mirror. "You shit," he whispered, "you got piss all over your arms."

The blond glanced down at his arms and the immaculate gauntlets that guarded them. Not a trace of yellow marred their shining perfection, and no liquid covered the swirling pattern that covered them. With a shrug he removed the steel protectors and ran his arms under the water. As he turned for a paper towel, one of his hands casually, almost accidentally, brushed against Jessie's crotch. The contact was feather-light, but Jessie felt his penis become immediately erect. He looked down at his pants, and the wet spot the blond had left there infuriated him all the more. He grabbed the boy's gauntlets and pretended to study them as he again brought himself under control.

"You shit," he repeated. "Where did you steal these?"

"They were a gift," the blond replied quietly. Had the boy seemed any less confident, his voice would have sounded weak and uncomfortable. As it was, it sounded as if the blond were stating a fact, a fact which precluded personal involvement. His gaze rested on Jessie's face, and Jessie found himself immediately unable to meet his eyes.

Staring at the gauntlets as he thought of what to say next, Jessie backed up against the door. "A gift from your mother?" he asked.

"From Louis Debris."

Jessie's gaze leapt from the gauntlets in the shock. Debris, front man for Last Despair, would never give anyone anything. "Bullshit!" he yelled. "Debris never gave you anything." He threw the gauntlets to the tile floor. As the blond bent to pick them up, Jessie reached out and put his left hand on the side of the boy's face. "Why did Louis give them to you?"

The blond straightened and shrugged. "He never said. I guess he liked me."

"Why would he like a shit like you?" Jessie demanded.

The blond reached up and took Jessie's hand, still resting on his cheek. "He found me ... different."

The boy slowly drew Jessie's hand across his face and brought it to his mouth. His tongue flicked out, quicker than a cat's, and licked the index finger. The blond's free hand reached around Jessie, slowly drawing the singer to him in an embrace.

Jessie found himself unable to resist or even to move. His left index and middle fingers were in the boy's mouth, and the hand the boy had used to guide Jessie's now reached out to the singer's shirt. Jessie felt his stomach muscles jump as the hand reached under his shirt and rested on his abdomen. The blond had finished sucking Jessie's fingers and was now gently licking the singer's arm. Then two hands took the hem of Jessie's shirt, and he raised his arms high as the boy lifted the shirt above his head.

Now the blond lowered his head to Jessie's chest, and Jessie felt teeth and tongue play across his broad pectorals. He reached for the boy's black shirt, but the blond angrily pushed his hands away. Jessie leapt backward as the teeth came down hard on his right nipple. The blond drew himself straight and moved close to Jessie again.

For the first time Jessie noticed that he was shivering, but he made no move to put his shirt back on. The blond reached his hands down to Jessie's still unbuttoned pants and slid one hand inside. Two fingers stroked the base of Jessie's penis and the other hand inched the singer's zipper down. His cock, freed from the constraints of the jeans, swelled further as the blond gently massaged it.

He didn't resist as the blond pulled him in front of the sink, nor did he seem to notice when the blond turned him around, one hand on his stomach and one on his side, so that his back was to the boy. He only realized what was happening when his pants lowered to the floor.

"Hey," he said as he looked over his shoulder, "I fuck you." He tried to speak with authority, but his voice sounded forced and distant. He rested his hands on the sink as the boy squatted down and stroked his legs.

The boy rested one hand below Jessie's balls as he used his other to lift Jessie's leg free of the pants. When his leg was clear, Jessie felt the boy's tongue run across his buttocks and rest momentarily in his anus. The same treatment rewarded the singer when his other leg came clear.

The blond rose behind him, running his left hand from Jessie's calf to the nape of his neck. The boy's right hand reached forward and wrapped around Jessie's cock. As he began to lazily stroke it, his left hand again traveled along Jessie's body, rubbing the singer's shoulders, caressing his sides and finally resting on his buttocks. The strokes began to quicken as Jessie felt the other hand begin to slide between the cheeks of his ass.

Jessie tightened his butt muscles and tried to move away, but the boy's grasp on his cock became firm and insistent. Caught and refusing to abandon the pleasure beginning to course through his groin, Jessie had no choice but to spread his legs wider as the blond probed his ass.

Each downward stroke on his cock coincided with the boy's finger penetrating his anus. Each upward one occurred as that finger came out. Together the two hands worked faster and faster, and Jessie also felt the leather of the blond's pants leg firmly against his bare thigh. Jessie closed his eyes and grasped the sink as firmly as he could, swaying with every movement.

Suddenly the boy stopped, and Jessie felt his legs almost buckle with disappointment. He opened his eyes and began to turn when he felt a hand crack down hard on his ass. "Keep facing the wall," the blond whispered harshly. Then Jessie heard the blond's pants unzip.

Seconds later the boy's fingers were again in the singer's

ass, and Jessie started as they applied something smooth and creamy to his anus. Then the fingers left his asshole and Jessie heard a short tearing noise as of plastic being ripped. He fought the urge to turn, and the boy's condom-covered dick began to pry his ass cheek's apart.

"Relax," the boy whispered in his ear. "Relax," he said again, drawing the word across his lips like a long and loving kiss. Then his cock began to enter Jessie's anus.

It seemed to take an eternity to fill him, and the time it took made Jessie more and more apprehensive. Despite all the men he had fucked, all the men he had forced to bend down for him, he himself had not been done this way since high school. What he remembered was the sharp pain as the older student thrust into him and the agony of the ramming that followed.

Now, however, it was more like the slow build up that proceeded a seduction, and Jessie gasped when the boy began to pull out. The blond did not withdraw all the way, however, and again Jessie squeezed the sink as the boy began to move back and forth within him. Immeasurably slow at first, and then faster and faster the boy began to rock against him. The pain was there, but so was an unfamiliar pleasure. Jessie began to tighten and loosen his ass muscles in time to the boy's thrusts. Soon his entire body was shaking, and somehow his prick swelled even further. Then the boy stiffened against him.

The cock plunged deep inside Jessie, deeper than ever before. He cried out, feeling his grasp on the sink begin to give way. The boy stood there, his penis slammed hard in the singer. His hands moved to Jessie's waist, holding them both firmly in place as orgasm shook him. Moments later he let go, and Jessie slumped against the sink as he felt the

143

penis withdraw.

Jessie turned weakly around as the boy pulled the condom off. With one hand the blond carelessly threw the rubber in a trash can as he steadied himself against Jessie with the other. Jessie stared down at the naked groin and legs, both far tanner than he expected, and felt the pressure of his own desire. Then the blond pulled off his own shirt, revealing his dark, slender torso, and kneeled in front of the singer.

"Thomas," the boy said, one slender hand moving up to cradle Jessie's testicles.

"What?" Jessie managed to stammer out.

"Thomas. My name is Thomas. Say it," the boy said. Then he brought his mouth down over Jessie's cock. His teeth barely touched the head before he engulfed the entire penis.

"Thomas," Jessie gasped out.

Thomas took his mouth away from Jessie's dick. "Say it again."

"Thomas," Jessie said, more firmly this time. Thomas again took Jessie's cock in his mouth and Jessie leaned back against the sink. He felt Thomas hum as he moved his head back and forth. Jessie's hands reached down to Thomas's blond head, spasmodically clutching and releasing his hair. Then Thomas stopped. His expression was as hard as ever, but for the first time Jessie saw a softness in his eyes.

"Again," he demanded.

"Thomas," Jessie blurted out.

"Say it again," Thomas insisted.

"Thomas. Thomas, Thomas, Thomas, Thomas ..." The last one came out as a scream as he exploded in Thomas' mouth.

"Thomas, Thomas, Thomas," he yelled as he felt the

semen shoot from his body.

"Thomas," he moaned as he felt the last glories of orgasm wrack his spine.

"Thomas," he whispered as he slid to the floor.

"Thomas," he prayed as he gazed into those cold, loving eyes.

"Thomas."

Althea Morin and I first hooked up because she met my friend Shariann Lewitt at a signing in New York. Morin publishes a sex magick zine called the Temple of Lilith. *She got the inspiration for this story when she went to an ultrahip fundraiser in the City where they had erotic cutting demos. "The Ceremony of Loneliness" explores something of the basic nature of sex, but it is also definitely one for you blood fans out there.*

The Ceremony of Loneliness
by Althea Morin

She stood with her arms flat against the wall behind her, the painted plaster throbbing with the beat of the music, damp and slick with the mingled sweat of bodies on the dance floor. It was as if she leaned against a thing alive, molding the skin of her back to an unyielding partner. She closed her eyes, lips slightly parted, breathing in the thick fog of the air, feeling the pounding thud of the bass in her fingertips, in the rustle of her hair against her cheeks, in the bones of her spine, in between her legs. The movement of dancers was a tangible thing, sound and rhythm, writhing, gyrating, pulsating. She was part of the wall, an unmoving bystander. With eyes closed, she felt invisible, a feeling either of safety or nonexistence.

Someone bumped into her, sliding sweat-slick down her side, falling laughing, "I'm sorry!", still entwined with some inamorata, also laughing on the floor wet with spilled drinks. Not invisible. She stepped over them to find some other part of the funhouse. A mirrored hallway. Another room. A stage. The music here hypnotic, trance-inducing, an arrhythmic wall of sound rising and falling with breath and blood in the veins. On the stage, three people lit by candles stood in a position of ritual. Two women and a man, the first woman bare-chested, a cross tattooed in the space between her breasts, the second woman tightly corsetted, blond hair piled high on her head, the man also shirtless, head shaved, tribal tattoos defining the contours of the muscles of his shoulders. The music rose in intensity, swelling like an adrenalized heartbeat, onlookers silent, still, all invisible here, as the corsetted woman moved to a

147

tray and selected first a shining steel pin a foot in length, facing the bare-breasted woman, who opened her mouth. The crowd fell silent enough that her sharp intake of breath was audible when the blond woman carefully and precisely pierced through both cheeks with the steel pin. Inches of shining metal protruded from either side of her face. One drop of blood grew and dripped down each cheek, only to be wiped away with a white cloth. She moved to the tray again, to select a scalpel-like blade. She turned her attention to the man. The woman with the pierced cheeks stood stock-still. With the precision of a surgeon, but with more sensuality than any doctor knows, the woman with the scalpel cut two intersecting incisions above each of the man's nipples. As she cut the man's flesh, the woman screamed, one scream for each slice, a high shriek. The metal rod visible inside her mouth shone in the candlelight. The blood flowed out, dripping around, then over his hardening nipples, down to his waist, where the dark fluid was absorbed by the cloth of his pants. The woman in the corset, her hair still perfectly arranged, stepped back, and nodded to the other woman, who, given this permission, went to her lover, bent down before him and began to lick the blood from his nipples, her tongue licking about the metal rod in her mouth, following the trickles of blood up his chest, licking the cuts themselves, both of their faces transfixed in ecstasy, the pain transformed to something more intense. Her arms went around him, holding him tight, bodies rubbing against one another, chest to chest, skin slick with blood. It was no longer a performance; the three turned to file off stage, the corsetted woman holding the tray of instruments, the other woman with her lover's hand in hers, his blood dripping down the cross tattooed between her breasts.

She watched, feeling her heart pump her blood contained by unbroken skin. She shook her head slightly, to free herself from the trance, looked about the room. She saw his eyes first, watching her steadily, as if he had been watching her for a long time. Why was he watching her, as if she were on stage, as if she were on display? The second thing she saw was that he was beautiful. From the curve of an eyebrow to the sensual line of his lips to the way his belt clasped with steel hooks around his waist, she wanted him, and lust hit her with a wave of confusion. Why was he staring at her? What had she done while she was oblivious to his observation? Had she been staring at the stage open-mouthed and drooling? Had her fingers moved to touch herself? Was it simply that her lipstick was smeared across her face? She realized that she was staring back at this stranger, and then she turned and fled.

She got lost trying to find the bar. Corridors twisted and turned into stairwells opening into other rooms, crowded with black leather, sweat and skin, music and conversation yelled above the unrelenting beat. She scanned faces, realizing she was looking for him again. Silently, she cursed herself for losing her cool, for turning and running the minute someone as much as looked at her. After all, why was she here, at this party alone? She knew what she wanted. Why had she run from it? Someone brushed against her shoulder. She jumped, and spun around, but no one she recognized was there. "Fuck! I bet he left," she mumbled to herself.

"You get ditched, baby? Why don't ya let me buy you a drink?" a guy in a beige suit and ugly tie leeringly slurred his words at her, gesturing at the bar, which was on the other side of the room.

"Fuck off," she muttered, and pushed her way through

the crowd toward the bar. Her money was in her bra, and she was trying to be discreet about fumbling in her shirt for it when she realized who she was jammed up against. The steel hooks of his belt were pressing into her hip. Her heartbeat caught and speeded. She couldn't get away this time. She had to do something, now. In the press of bodies she could feel almost anonymous, as if the hand which reached out and brushed fingers against the crotch of his jeans was not hers. It could almost have been an accident -- but an accidental touch does not linger, does not gently squeeze... She felt his flinching jump of surprise, the indrawn breath. She made herself look up to his face so close to hers, to meet his eyes with her hand still between his legs. Surprise, and recognition. His breath was warm on her lips as her fingers deftly twisted the button of his jeans open, pulled down the zipper, and drew out his cock, stiffening at the touch of her fingers, into the dark space between them. Just her fingertips, and the slightest touch of her nails ran up and down its length, then she grasped it tightly, feeling the blood surge into it, feeling it harden in her hand, the skin hot and silky-smooth. She glanced about- no one but he was aware of what she was doing. Someone roughly pushed by her toward the bar, and she was pushed up against her stranger. His cock was naked against her stomach, a softer pressure than the scraping of his open zipper and his belt. She wrapped her arms around his waist to avoid being separated by the shoving crowd, and she felt his hands on her hair, smoothing it back, caressing her neck and shoulders. His lips brushed her ear as he whispered to her, "Come with me, darling."

He pushed his cock back into his jeans, pulling his shirt down to hide the bulge there, took her by the arm, pulled her through the crowd, into a hallway, pushed open a closed door, and took her down a dimly lit stairwell, through another closed door into a small room filled with stacks of cases of liquor. Only then did he let her go, and pushed the door closed behind them. The beat of the music was now a muffled thump like a heartbeat through the walls.

She stood, leaning against the boxes, waiting for him to turn to her. He stood, facing her, saying nothing. She pulled off the short black tank top she'd been wearing, leaving her small, pale breasts exposed. Her nipples hardened at their new nakedness. She reached in back of her to unzip her shiny vinyl miniskirt, and pulled off that, underclothing and lace body stocking all in one move to stand in front of him completely naked. Her tattoo was now visible -- a snake, in exquisite detail, curled around her waist, its red tongue pointing down to that spot between her legs that she could feel pulsing, wanting to be touched. Her fingers trembled nervously, and she steadied them against her thighs. "So. Here I am. What do you want now?"

He looked at her and smiled. "What do I want? Would you do anything I wanted?"

"Maybe."

"Maybe not."

She looked at him, smiled, shrugged, half-turned away, almost as if she were not naked before a stranger. But her newly-bared flesh prickled in the unfamiliar air, and she could feel herself trembling- in anticipation or nervousness, she could not tell. She had not turned away too far to see when he moved toward her, his fingers reaching out to trace the coiled line of the serpent tattoo, down, sending chills along her back, down to the very end of the tongue, pausing, then running back up again.

"You didn't have to stop there", she whispered.

"Hmm? What if I wanted to? Maybe the question should have been, 'Would I do anything you wanted?'"

"Would you?"

"Maybe."

She moved closer toward him, one arm circling his waist, one hand tangling itself in the hair at the back of his neck as she guided his lips to hers, pressing her naked body against his still-clothed one, wrapping herself around him, wrapping her tongue about his, pressing close until there was no question of whose desires were to be fulfilled, or what those desires were. He lifted her, resting her ass on one of the stacks of liquor cases. She entwined her legs around his waist as he fumbled to free his cock from his jeans. She felt the hard pressure against her softness like a long indrawn breath of air never before tasted, sliding in . . . and then he was inside her, and his arms were around her, his breath hot on her breast, and the scent of his hair filling her lungs as they found their rhythm together. Sweat beaded on her skin as she moved to make the most of each of his thrusts, moving in syncopation with the thudding beat of the music from the dance floor above.

She found herself whispering, or perhaps she was not even whispering aloud, for her lover did not seem to hear her:

"This could be anything. You could be anything. The act is the same, no matter what trappings we choose to place upon it. Club, bedroom, motel room, the back of a van, or a starlit beach. You could be an anonymous fuck, a one night stand, a passionate affair, or my husband and the love of my life. This could be anything. We could be tattooed and pierced and dressed in leather and latex. We could play games of domination and desire. We could be naked and shy and unsure of what to do next. Anything could be next.

Any moment could be the end. Any moment could be the beginning . . ."

She felt his fingers intruding between their bodies, reaching down, feeling his own cock slipping in and out of her, rubbing her clit in rhythm with the motion of their bodies, and finally, as the contractions of orgasm began, washing over her like a flood tide, even her small gasping cries seemed remote, and finally there was only the moment, and there was silence.

This is another club pick-up tale, but with a genderfuck twist. L is the initial of a well-known DC scenester boy who fell off the planet a while ago. L, honey, give me a ring or drop me a line c/o Masquerade when you see this; the only folks who know how to get in touch with you are fat ugly goth kids who left their address book in their other enormous pants. Like the protagonist in "To An Excellent Slave", L might know how to work in an office, but L has no trouble getting the black lipstick and bondage gear right. None at all.

To An Excellent Slave
by L.

There have been times, like at this moment, when I think about the night I had met Evelyn and wonder where she is now. It's funny how in one night your whole life can be changed. For better, for worse, who knows and who cares? Me, I'm nobody. My whole life will be a figure, a number in some book. But Evelyn's life, she will burn an impression on everyone she meets and her legacy will live on in stories, like this one.

I had been working late on a project for Cynerdine systems. My job was easy, find bugs in the system and terminate them. It was around ten o'clock when I felt my mind begin to petrify and the words on my telemonitor began to melt into each other. I had to get out, leave, get my mind on something else. I decided to take a walk. I knew that around the corner from where I work was a club. I had passed it several times going home from work and never had the inclination to venture inside. I stood at the door and tried to talk myself into going in. "Work awaits," I said to myself. As I turned to leave I was stopped dead by a vision. Her appearance had struck me as a fantasy from some comic book come to life. A goddess, of six feet in height, with long jet black hair that fell to the top of her ass, long firm legs and generous bosom stood bent over adjusting the buckles on her knee-high boots. She said, "Going somewhere?" I had to say no.

I would like to describe her appearance. It was the appearance that could induce lust in any man, or woman for that matter, with a dark side. I found it to be somewhat more than any of my wildest bondage fantasies. She wore a latex corset. It accented the size and shape of her perfect breasts. I could see that her nipples were hard beneath. As I looked down, I noticed how tight her body was. She wore a black latex skirt that caressed her ass and beckoned you to touch it, with garters to hold up the fishnet stockings that showed off her long muscular legs. Her see-through raincoat enveloped the length of her, but I could see her beneath. I noticed the tattoo on her neck when she looked up to speak to me and I was intrigued. Her face had sharp features, yet the skin was so smooth, so soft. Her thick lips were covered by a lipstick the color of dragonfire that matched the color of her long nails. I noticed that all the rings on her fingers had sharp points. The kind that could hurt someone that touched her. Finally, she wore a variety of chains and bondage gear. I wondered if she used them. I saw the chain from her earring to her nose ring and I thought about how she must be a slave to pain.

Without a second thought, she took my arm and dragged me into the club. The club's name was Ground Zero. It was dark and the music was loud. As we entered I noticed how out of place I really was. There seemed to be a mass of youth lost in the angst of a society that had deserted them. They all wore black. Most looked terribly sad, or lost. Yet there was a dark energy that drove them into frenzies of "controlled" violence. I felt a sexual charge among these children of the night that I never knew existed. But, I saw young lovers as faces in the crowd and knew that tenderness wasn't a stranger to them, either.

Evelyn had a secret. Behind her dark eyes lived a creature of lust. I could tell by the way she danced that she knew how to use her body to its fullest potential. The way she caressed herself lightly, and the way her lips and eyes flared with the beat of the music made me desire her like the moon needs the night. I wanted her to draw me in and show me the ways of pleasure that I had never known.

She gave me a small tablet resembling aspirin. "Take this, you'll love how it'll make you feel." She placed one on her tongue and began to chew the pill. I did the same. She smiled and kept dancing. It tasted like shit. I thought I was going to vomit but I didn't want to lose face. I didn't want to reveal any weakness. "What is it?" I asked.

"It's X."

That was the last thing she said for a long time. I felt a wave rush over me. It felt so good. My body could feel everything around me, even the music. Then I noticed that my cock was bulging and throbbing within in my pants. The euphoria was unlike anything I'd ever felt. Visions of myself having my shaft suckled by this vampire filled my head. She danced up to me and started to rub my cock through my pants. "How do you feel?" she asked.

"Great, I feel great." I said this and I knew she could sense how nervous I was. She gave me a sheepish, evil smile.

"Oh," she whined, "How do you *really* feel? Do you want me? Do you want to feel me take you inside of me? 'Cause I want you." She laughed. I couldn't say anything. I didn't know if she was just teasing me or if she was really serious.

Before I knew it the music had stopped. The crowd slowly made its way to the street. I saw her talking to people and I was hoping she hadn't forgot about me. I felt kind of stupid not knowing anyone. She then turned and walked my way. "Hi, I'm Evelyn." Then she kissed me. The kiss was long and hard. I could feel her exploring my mouth with her tongue. "Hmmmmmm," she moaned. "I liked that. So what are you doing, now?"

"I don't know." I thought about the work I had upstairs and I didn't care. All I wanted was to be with her. "I'll go wherever you want me to." Saying that made me happy. Her response was another kiss. "My name is Kyle."

"Okay, Kyle. You are coming with me. I have such things I want to show you."

She took me to her apartment. It was an old warehouse flat in the wharf district. I knew right away she was an artist. Her work was mainly sculpture and sketchings of male and female nudes. The detail of her work was so realistic, I felt as if I was being watched as I walked into the open space. I looked closer at some the sculpture and noticed that some of the women had cocks and some of the men had vaginas. "Weird," I thought to myself.

"Take off your clothes, Kyle, and wait for me." So I did.

I waited, standing there naked, I thought about what this night had in store for me. Fears and joy made my head swell with anticipation of something wicked. After what I guess to be about half an hour she emerged from behind a curtain which concealed what I imagined to be her bed room and the vision aroused the most intense desire and lust I have ever known. She wore a black, tight leather corset with black garters and stockings. No panties. The sound of her stiletto heels upon the floor of the studio resounded in my brain. In one hand she carried a whip and in the other a tube which looked like toothpaste. Feeling scared, feeling light-headed, my cock began to pulse and I could feel the blood fill the veins.

"Amanda, please help our guest into the position."

Out from the shadows emerged another figure, she was different. She had the face of an innocent child and her hair was as red as hellfire. She, too, wore the same dark clothing as her mistress, yet as my eyes flowed down across her swan-like neck, around her firm bosoms, down to her crotch, I noticed she had a cock! Amanda was tall and had a firm build. I was curious to see what would happen next.

Amanda approached me and said softly in my ear, "Don't be afraid, we going to give you such pleasures, and we will take our pleasure from you." She took my hand and led me to a masseuse table. She instructed me to lay down upon it prostrate. Then she began to massage my skin. Caressing and gently rubbing my back, Amanda carefully rubbed me from head to toes until I fell asleep. It felt so good I couldn't help it.

I was awakened by a tickling sensation. Evelyn had been stroking my sides with a crop. "Wake up, Kyle, it's time to play." I noticed when I went to reach for Evelyn that my hands were bound. I tried to stand, but my feet were tied also.

"What are you doing?" I shouted. "Untie me right now!" I felt fear grip me and I didn't like how things were going.

"Tsk. Tsk. That's not how we speak to a Mistress, is it? You've been a very, <u>very</u> bad boy. Thus, I must discipline you.

Amanda! Gag him, and . . . give him the probe. I will await your call in the other room." She left.

Amanda came over and grinned sheepishly as I lay helpless.

I begged her and pleaded her to let me go. She just responded with a smile and shook her head no. She whispered in my ear, "Do you see this?", she held before me a rubber ball with a harness attached to it, " I'm supposed stick this in your mouth and gag you with it so that you can't say things that you might regret saying, however, before I do that, I'd like to stick this in your mouth."

She positioned her groin in front of me and I saw a

large cock standing erect before me, the veins pulsed and I could see the tip was wet with anticipation. It was kind of large, about seven inches long, and I freaked. She placed her hand on my head and slowly guided her shaft into my mouth. I found my self letting her do so!

At first, it was weird to have so much hot flesh in my mouth. I licked it and tongued it and felt that cock respond to my actions. This aroused me. She told me to suck her. She moaned, "Oooh, that's it, suck me....hmmm, oh yeah, do it." She began to fuck my face and to ram her cock down my throat. I bobbed my head for all its worth. I began to gag and instinctively I relaxed my throat to accommodate her member. "Ohh...yeah...hmmmmmmm, that's it, suck me, baby, do it to me little boy, make me come!" Her legs began to quiver and then her body. She squeezed her nipples tight and I could feel the veins start pulsing in her cock. Then she came. It was slow at first but then gobs of thick jism came out of her cock. She pulled it out of my mouth and creamed on my face. "Oh, baby, that was good. Hhhmmmmmmmmm." She asked me if I was thirsty and without waiting for an answer she pressed her breast up to my mouth and squeezing, milk came forth and poured warm into my mouth. She put the ball in my mouth and wiped the come off of my face. She left for about ten minutes and return holding the toothpaste tube.

"I have to give you your probe now," Amanda said with kind of childish voice. I couldn't see what she was doing. But all of sudden, I felt her fingers on my ass. Then she spread my cheeks apart. I tried to scream, but I was gagged. She held my ass cheeks open with one hand and I felt her smear some sort of gel on my crack and anus. It felt slippery. Scared, I tightened my virgin anus. I knew what was coming.

Amanda mounted the table. I felt the fronts of her thighs burn hot against the back of my own. She whispered into my ear, "this won't hurt if you relax and want to enjoy it, if you resist, I'll split you wide open." I tried to relax. She first stuck a finger inside me, then two. Then she pressed her cock against my virgin rosebud. Surprisingly, she gently slid her cock inside of me. It was uncomfortable at first, but then it felt kind of nice.

I enjoyed it. I moaned with pleasure. Her pace began to quicken. She started to plunge her cock inside of me. I could feel each ridge of her cock at the opening of my tract. She slid a panel out of the table and my cock dropped through it. She reached around and began to stroke my cock. It felt wonderful. She masterfully brought the skin up and down the length of my stiff shaft. Then, suddenly, she let go of my cock. She spread my ass cheeks and tried to go deeper than before. It was both pleasurable and painful at the same time. The she grunted and I felt her cock slide out and a few seconds later, I felt spurts of hot come fly onto to my back. My anus was contracting and expanding uncontrollably. Amanda dismounted and licked the come off my back.

By this time, my balls were more blue than the sky on a clear day. I wanted to come so badly. Amanda left and called for Evelyn.

Evelyn emerged from a room in the darkness. She came to me and stood before me like a she-wolf gloating over her prey. She unfolded one fist and said, "this is for you." It was an anal plug. She walked over to my ass and shoved it in. I moaned, again with both the sensation of pleasure and pain. She took off my harness and commanded me to service her hot snatch. She was already dripping wet. She turned me over and refastened the bonds. She then mounted my face.

She drove her pelvis into my waiting mouth. Her clit was hard and wet with her honey. I sucked and licked her tight little hole as much as she would allow me. You see, she was in complete control. She could come down to my mouth or raise her clit out of reach. She knew I was hungry.

"Amanda," she called, "get me a cock ring, I want to feel his cock inside of me." Evelyn dismounted my face and allowed Amanda to place the cock ring around the base of my cock and the scrotum sack. "I wouldn't want you to come before I did. It would be heresy." She laughed and strode over my aching member. She slowly lowered herself onto my cock. She was burning hot and ready to be fucked. I could feel how warm she was before my cock even came close to her cunt.

The way it she felt was pure, she was dominant to the extreme. As my cock entered her, it felt like warm silk, and a wave of intense pleasure enveloped me whole. I began to tremble. As Evelyn to bring me in as far as she could, I could feel her starting to squeeze and release my cock with her vagina. I had never experienced such control and mastery! She had Amanda come to suckle on her nipples and rub her clit while she rode me.

"Oh, that's a good slave. Let your mistress fuck you hard." She rode me like a horse. "Hmmmmm. Service me you little prick. Do it to your mistress. Do it." She then gave a gesture to Amanda. Amanda stood on a stool beside the table and shoved her cock in Evelyn's mouth. She sucked it while squeezing one of her nipples and rubbing her clit with the other hand. Her contractions became tighter. I wanted to come, but I couldn't because of the cock ring.

"Oh, Kyle, Hmmmmm, I'm going to come. Oh, ohh, oh!" She then took one of my nipples in her mouth and bit it till it bled. The pain didn't matter anymore. She came in waves. Trembling and shuddering with each. "Oh, I'm coming." She screamed and it resounded in the warehouse.

Then without a word she dismounted. Amanda removed my cock ring, and she and Evelyn proceeded to suck my cock. Within seconds, I felt my balls swell and I knew I would soon be coming. As they sucked and stroked me, I felt my orgasm begin. My body began to shake and my pelvis started to grind, then it happened. I began to shoot my come into the air. What seemed like gallons pumped out of my cock and onto their hair and faces. They continued to lick and suck my dry.

When it was over, they kissed each other passionately and then each kissed me. "You're a good slave, Kyle." They undid my bonds, but I had to lie spent on the table for a few minutes. I was led to their bedroom.

Through out the night we explored the realm of bondage and sex. They showed me such things I would have never known. At one point, I passed out from exhaustion.

When I awoke, I was back in my office asleep at my desk.

I thought that this couldn't be a dream, it seemed to real. Just then, the trickle of people coming into the office began. I quickly finished my project.

The day was long, and I felt exhausted. Near the end of the day, someone knocked on the door of my office. "Come in," I said.

"You Kyle McBaine?"

"Yeah."

"These are for you." The guy brought in a bouquet of black leather roses. I looked for a card. When I opened it, it read:

To an Excellent Slave.
Lustfully,
E. and A.

t.d.k. is a wonderful sexual predator. She has devised a Straight Girl Bisexuality Test which can't be beat. It has only one possible outcome -- t.d.k. is the babe for you. And it just about never fails. (Actually, never fails as far as any oral history I'm familiar with goes.) When her story "Private" first appeared in Blue Blood #1, *most DC scenesters immediately salivatingly knew who t.d.k. had to be, even though not all of them knew the name her mamma gave her. t.d.k. has a number of semi-obscene nicknames which she answers to. I think we'll skip those here though, just in case some local folks are still wondering.*

Private
by t.d.k.

Growing up I never thought I was the type to be the other woman... until I met you. You looked so hot that night, quite the "club kid". Your hair was pulled back into a pony tail, except for the back. The back was filled with tiny braids that brushed your shoulders. You wore loose jeans tucked into combat boots and a little black top. Did I mention that it was little? Over this you wore an oversized man's jacket. The skin across your abs was dark as if you laid out in the sun (leaving one to wonder if there were tan lines) and your smile was charming in a sweet, open kinda way . . . But it was your eyes that first seduced me, they were so hungry. They devoured me.

* * * * *

My first impulse when I saw you at Rhea's party was to touch you.

I want to touch you. I crave to touch you.

I want to cup your face in my hands, pulling you close to me. My lips press against yours, sweetly, tenderly and I kiss the corner of your mouth, the high of your cheek. Nuzzling your cheek, I would slip my hand into your hair, tighten my fingers, pulling ever so slightly and push you against a convenient wall.

My hands slide out of your hair and down your neck as I pull back to look at you. Your head falls back as my thumbs stroke under the curve of your jaw, leaving your neck open and vulnerable to my lips and teeth. I lean forward. You feel my breath against your neck. I feel your shoulder drop, stretching muscles taut, ready, waiting, anticipating me.

Lightly my lips touch your skin. You flinch as goose bumps spread across your body.

* * * * *

I first saw you at Rhea's party which was being held in a loft in the art deco part of town. I couldn't keep my eyes off of you. You were like a live wire that's best to be avoided at all costs and I knew that was what I had to do. You must have noticed my avoidance dance. As I was leaving and Rhea told me that you were going in my direction and that you were wondering if I could take you with me, I couldn't resist.

On the ride home you told me your girlfriend was out of town. When we reached your apartment and you asked me if I wanted to come up for some coffee, even though I don't drink it, I didn't even think to say no. I knew what I wanted...I want you.

* * * * *

You can feel my lips part against your skin, my tongue hot, wet, pressing into you. Slowly, I let my teeth come into play as they barely rest against you, scraping lightly as I kiss up and down the column of your neck with an open mouth, lulling you into a false sense of me teasing you.

My teeth barely rest against your skin, at first, as I grip the straining muscle between them. Your hands raise up and grasp my upper arms and your nails dig into me as I begin to bite harder and harder. My hands are at your waist, tightening, squeezing, stroking you in unthinking passion. I can hear your breathing deepen as you gasp for air as I dine on your throat.

* * * * *

I was wearing a white blouse with ruffles everywhere and over that I wore a black bolero jacket. As I closed the door to your apartment I wanted to take my jacket off but I couldn't move. When your hands raised to my lapels and pulled my jacket off of my shoulders for me, I sighed a silent sigh of relief. Tilting my head back you placed your mouth on my neck as I felt your teeth against my skin I couldn't help but shuddering in pleasure. My jacket dropped to the floor and your hands went to the buttons of my shirt. I wanted you to rip them open but no, you were a slow tease all the way. As my shirt opened I could feel your hands accidentally brushing against my breasts, causing chills to shoot through my body.

* * * * *

I raise my hands to the buttons of your shirt and make short work of them revealing your body to my eyes. I start at your hands and stroke upwards until they rest on your shoulders. One slips under your shirt and cups the top of your shoulder blade. The other rests its palm over your heart, feeling its heavy beat increase under my touch. I smile in satisfaction.

I push your shirt off your shoulders. It falls down your arms and I hear the soft sound of fabric landing on the carpet. Trailing down your arms, my hands follow the path your shirt took. Grasping your wrists, I raise them above your head. My hands repeat their actions, this time stroking the underside of your arms, downward until my fingers brush your nipples.

They tighten in response. Cupping your breasts, I lean forward and kiss your darkened peaks. I lick them... swirl them... lave them... flick them... and wet them with my tongue. Pulling back, I blow on them gently. You moan and again I smile in satisfaction. You bring me such pleasure.

As my shirt slid down my arms I felt a shiver go through me. You caught my eyes with yours and as your hands tightened around my wrists and you raised them above my head I felt all control leave me. I am yours.

Your eyes go to my breast and I can feel it tighten in anticipation of your touch. I arch towards you and my hands lower themselves from the wall and my fingers bore into your hair as I feel the heat of your mouth. Pulling you to me I moan, deeply. Arching and twisting, trying to get you to take more of me into your mouth.

You stop and a whimper breaks from my throat.

As I raise myself from my half bow to capture your lips with mine. I let my hands drift down to the opening of your pants. They unbutton and unzip at an unhurried pace as I tangle my tongue with yours. I moan into your mouth as you slide your tongue against mine. My hands go to your hips and push your pants to your thighs. You shift your legs for me and your pants fall down around your knees.

Your shoes slip off easily and so do your pants. I kneel at your feet (blessing the decadence that leads you not to wear underwear) to remove them. Picking up first one foot them the other, I caress your heel, the sole of your foot, and your toes. I wonder briefly if it tickles at all.

* * * * *

As you look into my eyes my lips part. Please kiss me. I don't know if I said it out loud or not but luckily you know what I want. Your lips take mine. Slowly the tip of your tongue enters my mouth. Thrusting lightly

and sliding against mine as you fill me more and more. I moan as thoughts of you fucking me cram my brain.

* * * * *

I look up at you from the floor where I'm crouched before you. Looking, seeing the fluff of hair at the apex of your thighs (which cries for my fingers to tangle and delve in), your belly (where my tongue will dance), your breasts (with your nipples dark and tight), your mouth (moist and flushed with passion) and into your eyes (deepened with the passion between us). You are exquisite.

My hands slide up the insides of your thighs. My thumb barely strokes you. You tense. My fingers part you and find you slick with desire. I lean forward and the scent of you fills me. My lips part in anticipation. You can feel my hot breath against your tender flesh. Your body arches towards me as you clench your hands in my hair, pulling me closer, but I stop just short of touching you. Torturing both you and me. Delicious isn't it?

* * * * *

As you take off the rest of my clothing my whole concentration is directed at one spot. I ache. One entire area of my body pulses to the beat you dictate. Every breath you take . . . every exhale is felt. Anticipation fills me . . . consumes my thoughts. Makes me helpless. I want you. At this moment there is nothing I will not do for you. I am wholly and utterly yours. Please kiss me. Please . . . please . . . My breathing has become labored. I can hear myself as if far away. Touch me . . . anything . . .

* * * * *

The heat of my tongue dashes against you as I kiss you tenderly with my open mouth. Your gasp for breath screams "Finally!". My tongue delves into you as I spread your thighs wider.

One of your hands tightens almost painfully in my hair and the other tries to clutch on to the wall. Finding no purchase you moan "Please" to me. I know what you want. I lick you slowly. Your breath catches in your throat in almost a sob. You pull me tighter to you. Can you feel me smile against you?

You sigh as you feel my fingers brush against you and you part your legs for more. You are so wet. I could drown in you. It would be my delight.

* * * * *

I feel the heat of your mouth against me and I almost sob in relief. I spread my legs wider to make it easier for you to eat me. Oh God! Anything... I can feel your fingers tickling me behind your mouth. Please . . . Slowly they slid into me. So slowly . . . Don't torture me . . . No do torture me I love it. Slowly I can feel two of your fingers fucking me, sliding between my lips, rubbing against the smooth walls of my flesh as I try to grab hold of them. I can feel you laugh against me. All of a sudden you stop. No! Please! I cry your name out loud. Just as quickly you begin again, this time fucking me with increasing speed and strength. Ohhh . . . Yes . . . Fuck me . . . Ohh . . .

* * * * *

My fingers slip into you easily. I can feel you tighten around me. I moan in appreciation. You laugh silently. Tightening again and again around my fingers. I do so love

171

it when you do that. I thrust into you with tiny motions as I let my tongue tangle in your curls. If I pull out now will you miss me?

I pull out suddenly and still my tongue. You say my name in such an enticing way, but that's all you say, because I find I can't resist, I must be inside of you. I thrust two of my fingers hard into you and you cry out with pleasure. Again and again I thrust into you fucking you harder and harder. I can feel you trying to grasp hold of me tighter and tighter. Squeezing me to my rhythm. You are mine.

This goes on until, accidently my teeth bump you and this seems to trigger your orgasm. Your thighs tense and begin to tremble. Your breathing has become ragged gasps for air and you pull me ever closer to you forgetting all thoughts of propriety as you bump and grind faster and faster, clipping yourself against my teeth and tongue.

* * * * *

ohyesohyeslickmebitemeswallowmefuckmeharder. . . harder . . . anything . . . anything

* * * * *

I take off my clothes and lay next to you on the floor. As I embrace you and smooth your hair, you kiss the last of you off my mouth. And as you nuzzle my breast, I can hear you murmur, "When will she be back?"

Yon Von Faust contributed this story to Blue Blood #2, *along with an interview with Poppy Z. Brite. He has done endless band interviews and his writing can be found in a number of other magazines, particularly those of the Gothic persuasion, including* Propaganda, Isolation, *and* Cyber-psycho's A.O.D. *De-Compression Press recently published* Wicked Dreams, *a collection of Von Faust's short work and poetry. His novel* Sybaritc Vampire *is expected out in early 1997. And, okay, it is possibly conceivable that Von Faust might be a kinky boy who is genuinely into erotic cutting and maybe this is another one which is not too incredibly fictional. Possibly conceivable.*

Lacerations

by Yon Von Faust

The urge strikes intermittently, sometimes lying dormant for years, other times rearing its head daily. I can't control it, I don't want to. It is more of a need than a feeling or craving. A need that must be fulfilled. The lust for blood.

The taste of my blood, I like it. I've always correlated love and pain, the two feelings which dominate and are inextricably entwined in my psyche. This unnatural association, and I know it's unnatural although I have no delusions that I am a vampire, combined with 25 years of disillusionment in western societal values and mores, makes me believe that there is nothing wrong with my source of release . . . Bloodletting.

The taste of my own blood always brought forth a wellspring of memories. Childhood, the taste of my own blood as I would mercilessly pull my own teeth in hopes of a visit from a Tooth Fairy that never came. Adolescence, fighting with other disenchanted youths, getting the inevitable bloody nose and tasting the crimson flow as it spilled onto my upper lip and into my eager mouth. Adulthood, working on numerous construction sites, slicing my hands to ribbons and sucking on the warm bloody digits, enjoying the salty taste of my life's elixir.

After being unemployed all summer, I jumped at the opportunity to work at a record warehouse in mid town Manhattan. The job was great, but things at my apartment were not. My room mates were driving me insane, or was it sane? They would constantly bombard me with their shallow mainstream ideals, encouraging me to shed my alternative lifestyle and appearance and be "normal".

Not long after my relocation from New Jersey to New York, my need, and depression began to manifest. Loneliness and despair followed me like faithful dogs through out my daily existence. Apathy towards everyone and everything enshrouded my soul, I was emotionally numb to the world. It was this apathy, combined with the need for some sort of feeling, that caused me to once again indulge in the act of bloodletting and self scarification.

On the night of the September 1990, Danzig show at the Beacon Theater, my need reached it's peak. I had to bleed, I had to suffer. My soul needed to be purged, my body cleansed.

The half case of beer I drank, along with the two and a half packs of chest kickers I smoked before entering the theater left a fetid, decayed taste in my mouth. Initially I was entranced by the music, but as time wore on my mind wavered. I walked out into the lobby for another smoke and a brew. As I reached for my cash to pay the attractive barmaid, blonde hair and jutting cleavage, nipples clearly visible through the fishnet shirt, my index finger was neatly sliced apart by the box opener I had inadvertently pocketed from work. It was just a single edged razor encased in a fancy metal casing, but it did the job.

The cut was bad enough to warrant stitches, but until I pulled the sliced flesh apart, it was not bleeding at all. Once the flesh was separated the blood flowed copiously a tiny river of crimson running down my finger and into my palm. I held my hand palm up, so I would catch the crimson flow and cause it to pool. The desire became too much and I tilted my hand towards my face, mashing my palm up against the parted lips and crooked teeth. Instead of relief, my hunger grew, and much to the apparent revulsion of a few fashion

Goths, I once again separated my skin this time I directed the crimson flow into my beer. The taste was unique, but pure undiluted blood was what I genuinely craved. After chugging the mixture down and crushing the smoldering chest kicker under my heel, I pursued my goal. I needed blood, Fresh Hot Blood. Pain. My pain.

I returned to my seat, tuned out my babbling friends, the screaming crowd, and the crushing metal guitars. I wanted pain and blood. I was numb both my body and soul were numb. I had no feeling in my arms or legs. The pain would remind me, prove to me that I was still alive and that this insanity called life was not just some horrible nightmare.

I pulled out the cutter and scoffed at the warning "Caution Razor sharp". I lifted my sleeve and cut slowly relishing as the cool steel slid across my tender flesh. There was no agony, only a feeling that transcended pain and was merely sensation. I could see the skin separate as the blood came to the surface and flowed in rivulets down my biceps. I watched it flow for a moment or two before flicking out my tongue to sample the salty iron like taste of my alcohol sodden blood.

Instead of licking the blood from my flesh I was now sucking with all the fervor of a piglet at it's mothers teat. I was so enraptured that I was unaware of the lack of music and the dissipation of the crowd. My friend nudged me and I pulled my mouth from the wound. I noticed the topical hemorrhaging around the self inflicted wounds and smiled. I needed more...

The keen interest I held for my hemophilia now flickered like a timid specter. Always totally out of my control, It would disperse as abruptly as it manifested. It coalesced when I met my lover, after a bit of small talk I knew our tastes would mesh...

Among other things, we shared similar musical tastes, mode of dress, delight in chemical alteration, and above all a penchant for blood. Upon meeting her I thought perhaps she might be a true vampire, for I did believe in these creatures, but now I have my doubts. From the inception to the demise of our relationship we shared 12 episodes of erotic bloodlust.

It was a cool, crisp, Autumn night, the smell of wet decaying foliage had not yet chased the clean crisp summer air into hiding. It was Friday, and I was heading out to Long Island to see my lover. My heart and mind were racing in anticipation of what was to come. I smoked a chain of cigarette after cigarette while I sped along trying to pass the time, my customized Black VW beetle roared noisily through the contrasting silence of the deserted Long Island highway.

Having reached my destination, I entered my lovers abode. The rural sounds of the night added to the ambiance created by the morose songs on the Full Gothic Jacket compilation tape, and the medieval melodies of The Dead Can Dance. The lava lamp on her vanity bureau cast a red glow evocative of burning embers, adding to the bestial cave like environs of her curtained boudoir. The undulating wax suspended within the lava lamp looked like blood emerging and merging, in the free fall of deep zero gravity space.

As we embraced, my lover, nuzzled in the crook of my neck whispered "I'm thirsty", and bit into the hot delicate flesh. As she pulled her mouth away I tentatively placed my hand upon the swelling bruised flesh. Emotions of shock and arousal commingled and became virtually indistinct. We embraced again, the shadows from the lava lamp and the numerous candles placed around the bed cast dancing shadows across the ceiling. My heart was rapidly beating in anticipation of the first cut, the feeling of my flesh disgorging it's ruddy elixir into her warm receptive mouth. I thought about the act we were about to engage in. Blood letting. Not the type of blood letting one does as a child to become blood brothers, or to sign some secret pact that is soon forgotten. We were about to release copious amounts of my blood for her enjoyment, to fulfill her craving for blood, and my masochistic tendencies. I needed to bleed, I needed to feel my nerve endings scream in pain. I needed to feel the sensations of my flesh being torn and I needed to feel my hot blood flow across my body. I deserved to suffer, to be deprived while she dined upon my blood. I had earned the right to suffer at her hands.

Slowly disengaging myself from her embrace, I sauntered over to her desk. Here, the accoutrements which would allow our ritual to commence were laid out before me like a surgeons tools. I would use these various items to divert the flow of blood from my bodies fleshy confines and into her eagerly awaiting mouth. As I sterilized the double edged razor blade, first in flame, then in an alcohol saturated cotton ball, I felt the chemicals we imbibed earlier in the evening begin their work. My perception started to alter, my senses became even more muddled, ever more dull, the need to feel anything, something, on the somatic level became an almost unbearable hunger. I was numb.

She wrapped her arms around me as I made the first of many incisions that night. Avoiding the jugular, I managed to deftly slice my neck wide open, the flesh separated as soon as the now warm steel brushed across it. The somatic sensation was over too quickly, I was denied my pleasure, I did not feel the pain. I knew I would have to continue to cut again and again until I was able to feel the incision and the ensuing pain associated with the separation of flesh.

I sliced again as I watched her reflection in the mirror. Her eyes were riveted on the tiny steel blade as I pushed it deeper into my flesh and freed more blood from my body. After the second deft cut, she tastes my blood. I watched as she eyed the blood trickling down my neck and forming a small pool in the crook behind my collar bone. I shuddered as I felt her hot breath along the length of my neck, tongue tracing the path of the blood. After what seemed like an eternity she placed her mouth upon the wounds to sup upon the blood now flowing freely from my body.

The blood always flows despite the depth of the cut. Although the amount of blood pleases her, the lack of pain disappoints me. I am not content with the incisions. Once again I release myself from her embrace and begin cutting repetitively. I can't feel the pain, yet the blood begins to flow from various 2 to 6 inch slices I randomly place across my well muscled torso. After a number of cuts, I begin to feel the pain that I deserve. I bleed the way I deserve to bleed, and as the pain receptors begin to awaken I continue to cut. I don't stop until the pain has grown from a tiny annoyance to the source of all my attention. At that point I can no longer contain my desire nor deny the tumescence that is now swelling in my loins.

We moved towards the sounds of Sativa Luv Box flowing from the speakers hidden under the raised bed. Our clothes quickly discarded we lay naked together. I rolled onto my back and pulled her short frail frame on top of me. She smiled as I bared my wounded neck and blood stained chest to her. Before bringing her mouth to mine she smeared the blood flowing from the various wounds across my bare chest then brought them to her mouth. I watched in rapt delight as she licked the blood from her gory digits. Without warning she latched herself to the wounds on my neck and began consuming the torrent of red liquid.

With feline fluidity she then brought her crimson stained lips to mine. I parted my lips to receive her and she let go with a torrent of blood allowing it to spill from her mouth and into mine, I had earned my reward. Our mouths sealed together I can taste my blood in her mouth as we explore each others orifices with lolling tongues. She maneuvered her body and I slid into her with all the ease of a hypo into a junkies thirsting vein, the consummation of our blood lust was now complete.

Blood and sweat mixed as our rhythm escalated. I began to feel as though my body and mind were no longer my own. I thought about a friend who had warned me about my blood lust and my desire for pain. He told tales of demons and spirits waiting to consume my soul, stating that bloodrites and self inflicted wounds were often open invitations to demons. I was too consumed by lust , desire, and the need for somatic feeling to stop the rhythm and end our dance of bloody passion. Even as the blood dripped onto the sheets, leaving red splotches which rapidly grew in diameter, she continued drinking from my wounds. She would move her mouth across my torso stopping at each laceration just long enough to obtain a mouth full of blood.

After our sexual release, we continued to remain entwined like two vines of Wisteria. The scent permeating the room was almost intoxicating. The smell of blood, sweat, semen, and human musk mingled with the frankincense and myrrh burning across the room on its bed of coal. We lay, completely satiated, bathed once again in the crimson glow from the lava lamp, and my blood, as the sun began to erase night from the sky and sleep enshrouded us like a dense New York City fog.

Until recently, Shariann Lewitt wrote under the name S.N. Lewitt with N standing for No Middle Initial. It seems her last publisher didn't think Lewitt's readers would believe a girl could know her science. But with the success of Songs of Chaos *with its high tech space setting and lesbian protagonist, along with a switch in publishers, it was deemed that Shariann Lewitt was worth her whole name. Although "Pipe Dreams" is a ghost story, most of Lewitt's writing features serious hard science; the tormented hero and counterculture lifestyle, however, are both constants in her work. "Pipe Dreams" appears in* Blue Blood #5 *and Lewitt also contributed short fiction to* Blue Blood #1. *Her short works can also be found in* Absolute Magnitude/Harsh Mistress, Newer York, *and various and sundry other magazines and anthologies. Check out her new hardcover* Memento Mori *plus her novels* Blind Justice *and* Cybernetic Jungle, *the latter of which is based partly on a live-action roleplaying game she was in and partly on a group house in which I resided. For the record, Lewitt does not just talk the talk; she is very active in the DC-Baltimore SM/leather scene and she has the best hand-worked iron bed on the planet.*

Pipe Dreams
by Shariann Lewitt

The curl of blue smoke reminded him of the stage, but this smelled saccharine-bitter while the dry-ice machine filled a club with a wet biting acid stench. This was only one more stage, no more. And Tim McKeon had been on enough of them he reminded himself, toured Europe and the whole U.K. and North America.

He shouldn't be afraid any more. The necromantic ritual to call up the ghost of his favorite writer was really just the creation of his imagination. There wouldn't even be a crowd watching. Not like when he played death music in the late night clubs for children with white painted faces and black-rimmed eyes, when he was somewhere between god and angel.

This was just one more piece of spectacle, cribbed from a book about ritual magic he had picked up more to impress people at the club than to actually read. But maybe the whole occult ceremonial would be the stimulant to get his subconscious on track on time. Something had to help. Nothing else had, not the quantities of gin and good hash, not the day trips from London, not the endless hours in the gym.

There was the room ready with candles and incense already burning, draped with black cloth and the altar fashioned after the one he had seen at Jimmy Page's house Boleskin. The house Page had bought because it had belonged to Alister Crowley. In fact, it did not look so different than the set for the past two videos he'd done, both the MTV version and the one that was too racy for the telly but was well received in the clubs.

They expected this of him. It was just one more element of the collage that went into the product called Tim McKeon. Even outrage had to be calculated. Though this time there was an edge of desperation behind the facade, a purpose to the personal theater. This next album was crucial and he was frozen. The music wasn't there. The words were mud. Nothing was happening.

Unlike his fans, Tim McKeon wasn't exactly certain that there was any supernatural. But he had read enough to believe in the suggestibility of the subconscious, which was where the music came from. If going through this little act stimulated his ability, unfroze the core that he couldn't touch, then it was more than worth the charade.

And it would help his credibility, to add oblique references to calling up the shade of one of his favorite authors to help him out. His fans would believe it. He made certain to appear the metaphysical high priest in all his public dealings. It was in his bio and his publicist had coached him how to hint carefully around the subject in the interviews.

McKeon took another hit off the elaborate antique water pipe. Like the ritual, this was expected. Fortunately, this was one of the requirements he enjoyed. Drugs, sex, rock and roll. The clean and simple things in life, not all bound up with the dark and twilight. Though it was the dark that he loved more than the simple.

Two more deep breaths of the saccharine smoke, three. It was just another kink in the corkscrew life-mythos of Tim McKeon, modern high priest of Dionysus. He couldn't admit he was afraid that even this extreme measure wouldn't work. That no matter what he did there would be no new album and his whole life and career would be defined by three years and seventeen songs.

Abruptly he put the pipe down. He left the sitting room and went into his bedroom, stripped and pulled on a single garment of black silk. Against the fabric his hands were dead blue white like a cadaver. The scent of frankincense and sulfur and balm of Gilead clung to the robe from his previous experiments.

He needed the help and he couldn't admit it to anyone. He had told the others that he was spending the day working on new lyrics for the album, the one they were due to start recording next month. And he didn't have anything at all. The well was dry. He was burned out, couldn't write.

The band was just on the verge of a big break. The last two indie albums had done exceptionally well, they were a cult item at home and were starting to sell in the States. The A and R person at Capitol was excited about them, pitching them in the industry as the next big and coming thing. Said he expected music that would shock the world in this next album, said that in some future of the universe this would be important music.

So Tim McKeon knew he had to deliver important music, and knowing that had made life strangely miserable and gray. Even drunk or high he couldn't escape the knowledge in the back of his head. He had to deliver on time, and there was nothing in him. Nothing at all.

The house was silent. Andrew and Gordon were out doing the bars and clubs on King's Road. He'd kicked out the pale, anemic girl with the faintly German accent he'd found in his bed when he woke in the early afternoon. There wasn't even any music from all the speakers wired into every room.

Only breathless anticipation coalesced around him as he stepped into the prepared ritual space. Fear sent shivers of delight through him. He looked around one last time at the fabric draped walls, the altar with its bowl and razor and blood colored rose, the perfection of the whole area. As good as Boleskin, definitely. Better.

And on the altar was her picture. He had cut it out of a book when he couldn't find another. Those overlarge dark eyes and skin whiter than his own watched now from the altar space. She had been dead for a century. She was only the symbol for his own creative abilities, he reminded himself grimly. Just as her book had symbolized the act and the unconscious desires long before psychology tried to strip humanity of its dark and primitive belief. Her book had been perfect, she was perfect, both _anima_ and muse, calling that from his inmost being.

He picked up the sword, held it overhead and began the incantations in Greek. At least he thought they were Greek. He's spent enough time studying the book and trying out various portions of the ritual before actually attempting it.

Heikas, heikas este babaloi.

But the words didn't matter, only the performance did, and McKeon threw himself into the part the way he always did when he sang. All the way, one hundred percent, and if it killed him then that, too, was one of the pleasures that enshrouded him.

Because he had to believe. The primitive in him had to be called up, assuaged, pampered.

A tay Malkuth, ve Geburah, ve Gedula, le olam omeyn.

Sword extended, he cut a pentagram in the air and imagined it flaming blue. Like the gas hob, like the electrical wires crackling in a storm. The blue burned hotcold over the sword, up his arm like a good hit taking hold. It was strong this time. He'd done it right, really right, and that knowledge excited him far more than any of the girls he'd seen in the club last night.

The opening was finished. He laid down the sword and approached the altar. There was nothing in the huge blue book he had bought at the occult store in downtown York that gave instructions for what he wanted now, but all his doubts were gone. Instinct was his guide, the artistic intuition that somehow made the music work before.

Besides, he had set it up himself. Once he'd written a song about it, about blood and life and walking through the worlds. The fact that he had created a situation where he had to live in that, that teased at the edge of his awareness with the familiar taste of making songs. Songs that felt like clay in his hands, that he could shape but that had their own life and integrity, too. When he could find and express them the way they demanded, when he was flying. When he was creating the music that had taken him out of the ranks of the ordinary, the hopefuls and the bitterly lost.

He smiled and pulled back his left sleeve, then raised the straight razor in salute to the portrait. Like everything else in the ritual, the razor was beautiful. The handle was black mother of pearl and it was tipped in silver filigree. The blade was watermarked blue steel, shimmering like a samurai sword. He looked at the blade for a moment and tasted the fearlust and the power around him. Then he made three neat cuts across the inside of his left arm, matching the precise scars already incised in his flesh.

Blood dripped down his skin and he collected it into the bowl. Blue energy merged with the red and the bowl looked as if it were full of living fire. *The blood is the life.* Maybe it was Crowley who had said that. He wasn't sure.

There was a perverse excitement in the bleeding, in the incense and her picture and the glittering power that he commanded. He felt detached and floating, watching himself perform each gesture perfectly, each intonation without flaw. Only the energy here was focused and clean, not the screaming raging congregation in the pit, slamming and crushing the life from each other while they paid homage to their own violence.

The crowds had excited him. The blood excited him. The razor was sharp and at first there was no hurt at all, only the disconcerting feeling of the blade moving under his skin. His pain, when it finally came, was piquant and pleased him.

The bowl filled slowly. He didn't need much. When he had maybe half a cup he dropped his sleeve again and left the cuts untended. The photograph he placed in the bowl, bound with life, and raised the sword once more.

More words. Infinitely more words. He used only his right hand on the sword, commanding, his thumb hooked over the guard and placed directly on the steel. He had forgotten who had showed him that trick, probably one of the fever-eyed slamming legions who had invited him to partake of more intimate rites after the shows.

The first few years they were playing out he had done all the rounds. There were the witches, traditional and Gardenarian, the Golden Dawn revivalists, members of both factions of Crowley's O.T.O. fan clubs, and a single alchemist who insisted on drinking tinctures of plants and minerals and poisons diluted in pure vodka. Tim McKeon had participated with all of them, often invited to play a prime role. Everyone knew that McKeon was a magician. He had done it for the excitement, the theater. Even his publicist found McKeon a little too close to the edge for her taste. It was fine and well to cultivate the reputation in the Gothic subculture; it was quite another to insist on starting recording at the "correct" astrological hour.

But this time he needed results. It had never mattered before. Always there had been the audience, the fullness of the words and the delicious pleasure of going beyond the rational, breaking all the rules.

He lowered the sword and laid it carefully in place. Now he only had to wait. He sat down on the cushion he had stored under the altar, his eyes focused on the picture and the bowl, trying to focus on one desire. Her. Mary.

Concentration was difficult. His mind wandered off onto the song that was only half finished in his head, that he couldn't quite get to come together. Back, he forced himself. Think about Mary.

He had spent hours reading about her, even about the world in which she had lived. A world that thought of itself as upright and rational and godly all at once. A world that had had a Gothic movement all its own, where rebel anarchists and free thinkers and occult charlatans had inflamed the underbelly of the night. He found that world very seductive.

He forced his thoughts back to Mary alone. How she had twisted the creation of life into something dark and shapeless and mute, a monster that was his private self. She would not be horrified by the razor scars that striped his arms. In her soul she had scars to match...

But there was a change in the room. The bluish energy darkened into violet and appeared to hover over the bowl. Then it shivered once, twice.

Tim McKeon strained forward and blinked. He thought it might be his eyes, the drugs, the dim light. But something was happening and it was real.

Girlish laughter broke the silence. "It's only imagination," he heard a young woman's voice say. She laughed again. She sounded muffled, far away, lost in the wires of a transatlantic call.

Then he saw her. She appeared like a hologram made from the violet mist trembling over the bowl. She was not the way he imagined her at all, nothing like the portrait painted when she was in her middle forties, ten years before her death. Although the large, overly intelligent eyes were the same.

This was not the Mary-mother to whom he had intended to bring his sorrows. Instead this was the nineteen year old girl of popular imagination, the one who had run off with a poet to Switzerland and spent a summer on a storm-tossed lake, in a villa where Milton had once stayed. This was the Mary who still had her talent and her nerve, who was not afraid to look at the darkness in herself and display it to the world. Who had the words he couldn't write, the calm courage he needed.

She was him, a creature from the center of his own mind. A projection of the creative within him was the way he phrased it.

It was hard to believe that the creature that stood like a violet hologram, taking more solidity from the blood, was a creation of his own mind. She was not only far younger than he had imagined, but more beautiful as well. Her expression, reflecting the haunted nightmares of her psyche, was the one he had cultivated so carefully and so rarely achieved. And in her hands she held a long narrow pipe.

She puffed on it and then held it thoughtfully away. She looked directly at him, and those overly large, lipid eyes were alien. She measured him calmly. "I see an illusion," she said quietly. "I think it must be from within my own imagining, a man. But I think he must be myself, a piece of myself. From the opium."

"No," Tim whispered harshly. "You are my dream."

She cocked her head to the side, thinking. "No, sir, I do not believe that is possible," she said politely. "But I am not certain that you are myself, either. Or my self is bleeding and fearsome, and I do not believe that. Any more than any of us are fearsome, that is." She turned slightly and it looked to McKeon as if she were listening to someone speak. Her lips moved but he heard nothing, as if this part of the dream was barred to him.

"Tell me where you are," she said serenely.

"I'm in a house in London," he said quickly. "A small house near the London Dungeon."

She smiled. "I am familiar with that area. Although I cannot imagine how anyone could tolerate the constant stream of thrill seekers and nannies trying to scare their charges with implements of torture closed away in cases. I have not lived in London in a while. A friend of my father's has offered to introduce me to Society in the season there, but I have always managed to decline. The glitter of ball gowns and titles and vying for invitations is not to my taste. All that matters in Society is making an advantageous match. But, my demon sir, I believe in free love and the natural superiority not of the titled classes but of the creative mind."

"Yes," McKeon hissed. The wild abandon in her words was an anthem that echoed in his own soul, that made the ardent iconoclast in him quiver with desire. "But where are you, and how are you breaking those rules? Because I am doing it by summoning you."

She looked at him quite sternly. "You did not summon me at all," she said. "I smoked the pipe of my own will. It is a journey of discovery, of finding the truth behind the illusion. Though I am not certain that you are any more substantial or have any more truth than do I."

"You are at Villa Diodati on Lake Geneva, where Milton once stayed," McKeon said, almost languidly. "And one night you will tell ghost stories and all try to scare each other. And yours, Mary, yours will be the best. A hundred years after you're dead I will read your book and think of the infinite twistings of my own mind. And because you wrote it I will know that I am not alone. Someone else knows my secrets, my vices. Someone else did not find them too terrible. I am not the only monster."

"But the monster is innocent and beautiful," she protested vehemently. "It is the proper Society man, the doctor, who is evil."

A violet tinged hand reached out to him and her bottomless eyes showed only calm acceptance.

McKeon tasted the words with disbelief. He had been called beautiful before, but for his face and not for his deepest identity, the self that was too horrific to see in the mirror. But she *had* seen, the very worst, and there was only serene approval in her expression. And she had called him innocent. The depraved, created gothic hero tried to sneer at the word, and shattered.

"Then you think I ought to write it?" she asked.

"You must," he answered, startled. "If you don't then I won't be able to write anything either."

Her smile was grave. "Then we shall both write," she said. "It will be a sacred trust, an agreement. George and Percy do this often, have competitions as to who can compose a better poem about some subject. So you and I shall have a pact. I shall write the story for you. And you must read it and be a fair judge. Although, of course you are only an opium dream." She sighed and looked sad.

"You're the dream," he said, but already her image was fading, the violet fading, separating, and the solid three dimensionality dissolving.

He was aware of the room again. The candles were low and there was a draft coming in under the floor. His left arm ached miserably.

All the books he had ever read on the subject of magic insisted that he had to close the ritual space, no matter how spent it was. He skimmed the book, left it on the floor and picked up the sword again. The closing was almost identical to the opening. He had memorized most of that. But this time the movements felt flat and he was aware that he looked silly, saying words he didn't understand wearing what amounted to an expensive bathrobe waving a sword around. Tim McKeon swore he would never bother with this magic business again. Obviously it was a complete crock.

* * * * *

His arm was still sore when he woke up. According to the red LED on his clock it was eight in the morning. He groaned. The last time Tim McKeon had seen eight in the morning was when he had gotten lost on his way home from a party in the country and stopped at a local coffee shop for directions and ended up buying breakfast for half the room.

He must have fallen out right after the ritual and slept straight through. He was better rested than he remembered being in a very long time. Something, some weight or burden was gone. The ritual seemed part of the night before, a dream perhaps. He'd been toking up, maybe he had been high and imagined the whole thing.

He enjoyed feeling free, feeling alive this morning. He

took a shower, left his hair towel dry and put on a clean pair of black jeans. The day was slightly overcast, gray. It made him think of light on a lake, on silent deep water. Lake Geneva, Switzerland, where once three famous writers had spent a summer of wild abandon.

He went down to the basement, to the studio he had sent up. The studio he hadn't entered for nearly a year. His hands were flying over the keyboard and the words and melodies were thick in the air around him.

He completely lost track of time, until suddenly he realized he was screamingly hungry and went up to the kitchen. The clock there said it was ten at night. He hadn't noticed. He didn't care.

He brought some provisions down with him, a couple of tins of sardines, half a loaf of bread, two bags of crisps and a large box of chocolate biscuits. Then he went back to work until he fell asleep in the deep carpeting on the studio floor.

* * * * *

He dreamed of Mary. He had forgotten she was so beautiful, so perfectly serene and still like the grey glass water of the lake. Not his *anima* at all, but his muse. He had never had a muse before and suddenly realized that he was writing for her. Because he wanted to share it with her, because if she saw it then she would know that he was real and worthy, and she would smile at him. He was writing because he had fallen in love with her, with his idea of her. And she was more than a hundred years dead.

The truth did not stop the work, did not impinge on the fevered creativity. Everything and everywhere was music, songs that were impatient to be captured by his sixteen track, to be embellished and supported later with fine production and flawless craft. This was raw, new, but it was all of a piece.

He couldn't stop. The music was greater, stronger than he was. His own lust fueled it, every finished song was one more to play for Mary, to make her see him as himself. To make her love him back. The women he had known in their white face and black leather seemed only a pallid imitation of the deep core of brilliance and sadness that he had seen for those few moments in the opium dream. Maybe she wasn't always so grave, so gothic, maybe it was just another illusion. But the doubts were smaller than the songs.

Tim McKeon stayed in the studio for five days, emerging only to use the bathroom and get more food. He was down to the stale donuts when the jag finally ended. After five days he had written nearly seven hours of music, culled down to four hours and twenty minutes of which was positively earth shattering.

He called the guy at Capitol, who was thrilled. He called Andrew and Gordon, and they listened to his tape twice, silent.

"It's better than good, man, it's fucking insane," Andrew said softly after the second time. "I'm impressed. This is going to blow everyone away."

Andrew normally didn't get excited about anything. Tim was gratified. To celebrate they went out on the town, down to the clubs on King's Road where everyone wore black and the music was loud and harsh and the lyrics were all about death.

Tim stood at the bar, a beer in hand, and surveyed the scene. He'd practically lived in this place for weeks on end, he knew every one of the people here. They were dancing, sweating, trying to impress each other with their chatter, which was all inane. There was Lisa who danced the night to forget the days working as a hotel chambermaid, and Jay-jay who drank and looked cool to be more important than everyone else on the dole. There was Spider the bouncer who was bored to death and read historical romances perched on his stool near the door, and Bajit who walked up to every stranger in the place at least once and told them about her academic career.

It made him sick, suddenly. After the creative glut of the past days he could hardly bear the uninteresting sameness in the lives around him. He wanted to be out of here. He wanted to be in a villa in Switzerland with the Alps high all around, and have Lord Byron and Percy Shelley for conversation over dinner.

He left the club, waved down a cab and went home. The house was silent, almost comforting. He went in, dropped his leather duster on the first chair he encountered, and went to the living room directly to rummage for his pipe. He had to open at least three drawers in the living room side tables before remembering that he had stashed it in the kitchen under the sink.

It was an effort, but he took the large bubble-pipe upstairs to the room that was still set for the ritual. Week old blood clotted and congealed on the picture that had been cut out of a book. Tim looked at that picture and trembled. He had to get back to her. He had to give her the music.

He sank into the cushions and started up the pipe. The water like the blood was stale. It tasted gummy and the pipe took a long time to start. Finally he got it going. He took three, four deep hits off the pipe. It tasted foul, as if it had been left to lie more than a week. More like a century. And then the deep relaxation came, the false sense of drug-comfort that made everything sensuous and secure and perfect. Detached from the causality of daily life, he entered the illusion desperately, praying it was the door he wanted but strangely aloof at the same time. As if he knew, but was afraid of knowing.

He let the drug take him. The thick cushions on the carpet were like a pasha's palace, and he stretched out and felt embraced by oriental splendor. Coleridge had described it all so well. At a wave of a little black box he commanded the music on. It saturated his consciousness, as if it was in his head and his ears at once. He sank into the music until it filled his whole range of perception.

And then he saw her. Her long dark hair was free on her shoulders and she was wearing a white night dress with cascades of lace over her arms and breast like snow. White on white, innocent and unredeemed, predator and victim all at once.

She did not appear to notice him at first. She was seated on a large canopy bed with pages in front of her, reading them over feverishly. And then she looked up and met his eyes.

"It is not finished yet," she said gravely. "We have been so busy on the lake and there was the matter of Claire's pregnancy, you understand. But I have begun and am committed to finishing. Even if you are only part of myself, it seems you are a part of myself which must be obeyed."

"You must finish, Mary," he said softly. "We have an agreement, you and I. You promised you would finish the book for me. I finished the songs for you. Listen. I wrote it for you. Because of you."

She cocked her head and her mouth tightened into a line as if she were straining. "It is so distant," she said. "Like the thunder on the lake, like something from Hell. So perhaps when I think of you as my demon I am not so wrong."

"It'll go platinum," he said firmly. And then he realized that was not even close to anything he wanted to say. The words were all for her in the lyrics he had written down, the words that she could barely hear through the veil of a century.

"Please," he said softly. "It's my gift to you."

The music embraced them both, relentless rhythms driving it through them, primitive, free, abandoned and wild. Her dark eyes shone in the candlelight, tied and twisted on the bed, caught and pinioned and unafraid all together.

Then she turned as white as her starched lace. "But I was never gifted in music, I could not call up an illusion like this from my own mind. And you, you seem so very far distant and so real. But I cannot..."

He reached out, desire burning more sharply than the razor ever cut. He reached toward the white shadowed form, and for an instant he thought he touched cool yielding flesh. A lock of hair brushed his face and he was lost in the clean scent of rain.

"I love you, Mary," he whispered into her neck.

Ice ghost fingers snaked through his hair, traced the scars on his arms, on his chest. She leaned down and kissed the healing cuts he had made when he had summoned her, cuts deep enough that they were still black in the center and angry red across the white skin. She smiled at the self-inflicted injuries like a blessing, then shook the layers of downy lace away from her own sleeves and showed him neat white cuts that were more demure from being longer healed than his own. She looked at him, into him, and she knew him and took possession of his darkness. She enhanced it, reflected it like moonlight, like the black ink lake under the stars, like death.

For the first time Tim McKeon truly wanted to die. If

the deep slashmarks of his pain pleased her then he desperately wanted more pain. He wanted to fling himself into those consuming eyes and drown. He had given her his music, he had given her his soul and it was not enough.

And then it seemed that she was gone, or translated into the drug dream that followed. McKeon never was certain if the rest actually happened or was created from his own mind and the pipe. He thought he had used the razor again, her shining hands on his guiding the blade across both their bodies, pain and ecstasy burning together until the conflagration was all that was left.

Touch surprised him, and yet she was with him, here, draped across the heaped pillows like Coleridge's odelisque. But when he lay a hand against her knee he found flesh as cold as a November rain. As he lay simply looking into her face and wondering if he could get another key of whatever this was Andrew had sold him, she drew herself upright and leaned over him. She held a small knife in her hand, a pocket knife he didn't recognize. She touched the blunt edge to his cheek and traced the line of his jaw to his ear. Then he felt the point teasing across his skin, down his throat. Not quite cutting. Not yet.

Then she reversed the knife again and caught the blade under his tee-shirt. He felt the smooth safe edge glide down over his heard and across his belly as she cut the shirt to ribbons. She moved from his sight. He felt his boots removed, quickly, efficiently, and then the cool path of the knife as she slit his jeans up the leg, tickling his hip and slashing the waist. By the time she shredded the other leg and his clothes, now ribbons, fell between the cushions, he craved release.

The rhythms of his own music pounded in his ears, his blood. Always the blood. She sat on her heels and then moved over him, mounting him without revealing herself. He closed his eye for a moment to revel in the glory of sensation, feeding on it. But it was not enough. He needed something . . . more.

He returned his vision to her face. In her eyes he could see the mirror of his own, desire building in urgency but lacking. Needing. She arched her back and her hands fluttered to her hair. To the white rose tangled in the dark locks. She pulled it down and Tim saw the thorn-decked stem. She lifted just the fraction of an inch and slipped the stem between their joined sweaty thighs.

A sliver of pain pierced the frustration. Mary's lips curved into an incandescent smile. He could taste Paradise; he had never been so high, so torn, so utter sated and so deeply in need.

The razor was in his hand. Her cold fingers closed over his and she breathed in sharply. He used the razor again, her shining hands on his guiding the blade across both their bodies, pain and ecstasy burning together until the conflagration was all that was left.

But when he woke up amid the silken cushions on the floor he was sad and elated together. There was no soreness, though it seemed like a very old scar was traced across his body that he had did not remember.

* * * * *

The sun was setting over London in a glorious array of amber and pink haze. The stones of the London Dungeon were alternately gold and red as the sun stained them with oncoming night. Tim McKeon left his house and started to walk down the street, looking at everything around him as if he had never seen it before. He wondered it the antique shops and colorful but expensive dealers had clustered around the Dungeon waiting for tourists in Mary's London. Some of the shops looked like they might have been there that long.

Maybe it was just a play of light on the display window that attracted him, or the sense of time caught in the sundown in the little antique book shop near the corner. He turned in on impulse. The dark leather bindings with their ribs showing and gilt letters made him think of Mary, of her books. Though he had never been interested before, he went to the S's and began to browse the shelves.

The book nearly jumped into his hands of it's own accord, a first edition of *Frankenstein, or the Modern Prometheus* in the original binding. The leather caressed his hands like her pale flesh. He opened the book reverently. It was his, just as his music was hers, mutual muses through the pipe. No matter if she was merely a creation of his own desperation. She was and always would be his Dark Lady, the inspiration so perfect and glorious and pure that she could not possibly exist outside his own creation.

He looked at the yellowed page, and froze in shock. There, written in ink that had once been black but had faded to deep violet over the nearly two centuries intervening, was an inscription.

To the man in the pipe dream, though I cannot believe he really exists, I must express my gratitude and debt for the writing of this book. And for the echoes of the music of Hell that still sound in my sleep and the memory of a night with a demon lover who has never lived apart from imagination.
—Mary Wollstonecraft Shelley 1818

A few years ago, I first came across Poppy Z. Brite's work in a couple of semi-pro zines owned by an old housemate of mine. Since then she has authored three remarkable novels. I have never read anyone else's stuff that comes close to Brite's in communicating the spirit and feel of the Gothic subculture and that of other marginal folks. The following review is reprinted from Blue Blood #3: *"Plus, where her first novel* Lost Souls *was sexy, her new book* Drawing Blood *is downright erotic. Brite make her settings come alive with her keen perceptions of fine detail, but what I really love are her descriptions of cool alternative people, particularly pretty boys and their intimate anatomy. Never before has a penis been described as so beautiful:*

'The skin of the shaft was textured, slightly rippled beneath the surface. The head was as smooth as satin, as rose petals. Trevor rubbed his thumb across it, squeezed gently, heard Zach suck air in through his teeth and moan as he let it out. He could see blood suffusing the tissue just beneath the translucent skin, a deep dusky rose delicately purpled at the edges, crowned with a single dewy pearl of come. It was as intimate, as raw as holding someone's heart in his hands.'

Whether or not a particular passage is explicit, there is throughout a heightened sense of anticipation and lush sensuality. And the main characters are all wet dreams unto themselves. Eddy is the defiant Asian stripper with a zillion earrings and a quest for self. Zach is the vampire-complected philandering hacker boy on the run from the Feds. Trevor is the long-haired tortured artist returning to the haunted house in which his father murdered the rest of his family.

The spookiness is effective because of its sense of being almost familiar and because you hunger for the characters so much you can't bear the idea that they might not make it. We've got hot and cold running blood and semen and characters who remain hyper-productive, capable of growth, and creative no matter how much dope they smoke. All this and a gripping plot too. All right!"

Brite's short stories can also be found anthologized in the Swamp Foetus *collection, along with many magazines and anthologies including* Cemetary Dance *and Thomas Roche's* Noirotica. Exquisite Corpse *is her new novel published by Simon & Schuster and she is currently working on a biography of rock diva Courtney Love. The following story is not particularly erotic, but it involves the continuing adventures of Steve and Ghost, two of the coolest characters from her longer work. Plus, it was just so damn funny, I had to have it for that upbeat closing note. Nope, no gloomy readers here.*

America
by Poppy Z. Brite

The desert after midnight was an arid zone of silver and blue, the highway a glittering black ribbon into nowhere. The formations of rock and sand were incomprehensible to a Southern boy, wrong somehow, like the bones of the world showing through the desiccated flesh that was this land. Buttes. Dry lakes. Mesas. Who had ever heard of such things? Steve shook his head and took another hit off the sticky green bomber he was holding, and the desert went a shade weirder.

They had picked up a thirty-dollar quarter bag way back in Dallas, and it was so good it looked like it was going to last them through the next Lost Souls? show in Flagstaff. When your two-man band was touring the country in a gas hog of a '72 T-bird, when your household consisted of a guitar, an amp, a couple of microphones, a cooler, two backpacks full of dirty laundry, and a blanket stolen from a Holiday Inn, when you'd been on the road for upwards of a month, thirty-dollar bags of excellent pot were a small but welcome manifestation of slack.

Steve cocked his elbow out the window and leaned into the wind. His dark hair whipped across his face, five days unwashed and one year uncut. He could put it in a ponytail now, but he left it loose when he drove because he liked the feel of it blowing. He had a fresh sixpack of Bud on ice. There was only one thing wrong with his world tonight.

Ghost, curled in the passenger seat with his sneakers propped up under the dash, kept singing a toneless snatch of song under his breath. "Been through the desert on a horse with no name . . . Felt good to get out of the rain . . ."

Steve twisted the radio dial. FM, AM, it was all the same: dry scratchy static clear down the line, like the sound of the desert clearing its throat.

"Ain't no one for to give ya no pain . . . Nuh, NUH, nuh-nuh-nuh-nuh --"

"Quit singing that fuckin' song!"

"Huh?" Ghost looked up. The moonlight turned his eyes and hair paler than ever, turned his skin translucent, made him seem a true thing of ectoplasm, subject to shimmer and disappear at any moment. The open can of beer in his hand spoiled the illusion a little.

"You're singing that America song again. Quit it. I hate that song."

"Oh. Sorry."

Ghost shut his mouth and returned to whatever reverie Steve had dragged him out of. For thirteen years they had spent long easy stretches of time in each other's company. They had passed the last part of their childhood together, had grown up together. During these weeks in the car, though, their friendship had reached a new equilibrium. They talked obsessively and often, but they understood one another's silences too. Sometimes they went for hours without saying a word.

But once in a while they got on each other's nerves. A few miles later, over the roar of the slipstream from his cranked-down window, Steve heard, "Nuh, NUH, nuh-nuh-nuh-nuh . . ."

He gritted his teeth. He knew Ghost wasn't even conscious of singing aloud. Being a singer, Ghost tended to give voice to whatever scrap of music flickered through his brain. Sometimes it was unique and brilliant. Sometimes it was a glob of dreck from the seventies. America was only the first in a turgid alphabet soup of bands Steve hated, horrible bands with stupid one-word names: Boston, Foreigner, Triumph, Journey, Bread . . .

"Nuh, NUH, --"

"Guess you heard of the man-headed cat that lives around here," Steve said.

Ghost stopped singing, looked again at Steve. His pale blue eyes shone silver in the light. "The what?"

"The man-headed cat. It lives out here in the desert, eats horned toads and rattlesnakes and roadkill, drinks liquor from cacti. About the size of a bobcat, but with the head of a man, shrunk down like."

"Really?"

That was the fun of telling tales to Ghost: he was always prepared to believe them. Born and partly raised in the mountains of North Carolina, he'd seen and touched things as weird as any Steve could come up with.

"Sure, man. Way I heard it, this guy got lost real late at night and his car broke down. Not on a main highway but way the fuck out on some deserted track you can't find on the map. So he drank a bottle of whiskey he had with him and passed out on the hood of his car.

"When he woke up, the man-headed cat was sitting there watching him. There was a full moon shining off the sand and he could see it clear as day, the bald head and little wrinkled face. It had green eyes and the fur started at the neck, right at the collarbone. From there down it was all cat. But man-headed."

"Could it talk?"

"Shit, yeah! It could cuss! It opened its mouth and what came out was, 'Goddamn-shit-ass-mother-fuckin'-bitchofagoddamn-fuckin' --"

"Then all of a sudden it lunged and took off chasing him. They ran and ran out across the desert, so far that the guy knew he couldn't ever find his car again, so he knew that either the man-headed cat would kill him or he'd thirst to death out there. He figured it'd be better to go quick, so he stopped to wait for the cat. He was out of breath, exhausted; he'd run as hard as he could for miles.

"But when he turned around, there was the man-headed cat grinning and cleaning the sand off its paws. 'That was a nice little run we had,' said the man-headed cat. 'Motherfuckin'-piss-cunt-Jesus-lickin' --' Then it crouched down, and its green eyes glowed in the moonlight, and the guy could see hundreds of tiny sharp teeth in its grin . . ."

Steve stopped.

Ghost waited about ten seconds, his eyes wide, his fingers scrunching the hem of his T-shirt. "What did it do to him?" he asked finally.

"Nothing," said Steve. "A little pussy never hurt anybody."

Breinigsville, PA USA
27 September 2010
246218BV00001B/14/P